マニュアル改訂/作成にあたって・序文

1. 中枢神経
    1-1. 悪性神経膠腫
    1-2. 低悪性度神経膠腫
    1-3. 脳胚腫
    1-4. 髄芽腫
    1-5. 良性脳ına瘍 ………………… 6
2. 頭頸部 ………………………… 9
    2-1. 眼・眼窩腫瘍 ……………… 9
    2-2. 鼻腔・副鼻腔癌 …………… 10
    2-3. 口唇と口腔癌（舌を除く） … 11
    2-4. 舌癌 ………………………… 12
    2-5. 上咽頭癌 …………………… 12
    2-6. 中咽頭癌 …………………… 13
    2-7. 下咽頭癌 …………………… 14
    2-8. 喉頭癌 ……………………… 14
    2-9. 耳下腺癌 …………………… 15
    2-10. 甲状腺癌 ………………… 16
    2-11. 原発不明の頸部リンパ節転移
        ………………………………… 16
3. 胸部 …………………………… 22
    3-1. 乳癌 ………………………… 22
    3-2. 非小細胞肺癌 ……………… 23
    3-3. 小細胞肺癌 ………………… 24
    3-4. 胸腺腫・胸腺癌 …………… 24
4. 消化器 ………………………… 30
    4-1. 食道癌 ……………………… 30
    4-2. 結腸癌 ……………………… 31
    4-3. 直腸癌 ……………………… 31
    4-4. 肛門管癌 …………………… 32
    4-5. 原発性肝癌 ………………… 33
    4-6. 胆管癌 ……………………… 34
    4-7. 膵癌 ………………………… 34
5. 泌尿器 ………………………… 41
    5-1. 膀胱癌 ……………………… 41
    5-2. 前立腺癌（外照射）………… 41
    5-3. 精巣腫瘍 …………………… 42
6. 婦人科癌 ……………………… 45
    6-1. 子宮頸癌 …………………… 45
    6-2. 子宮体癌 …………………… 46
    6-3. 膣・外陰癌 ………………… 47

    8-3. 上大静脈症候群 …………… 56
    8-4. 脊髄圧迫 …………………… 56
9. 皮膚癌 ………………………… 60
    9-1. 皮膚悪性黒色腫 …………… 60
    9-2. 基底細胞癌・有棘細胞癌
        （扁平上皮癌）……………… 60
    9-3. メルケル細胞癌 …………… 61
    9-4. 血管肉腫 …………………… 61
    9-5. 乳房外ページェット病 …… 61
10. 骨軟部腫瘍 …………………… 64
    10-1. 骨腫瘍 …………………… 64
    10-2. 軟部腫瘍 ………………… 66
    10-3. 切除不能骨軟部腫瘍 …… 66
11. 小児 …………………………… 69
    11-1. ウィルムス腫瘍 ………… 69
    11-2. 神経芽腫 ………………… 70
    11-3. 横紋筋肉腫 ……………… 71
12. 良性疾患 ……………………… 74
    12-1. 脳動静脈奇形 …………… 74
    12-2. ケロイド ………………… 75
    12-3. 甲状腺眼症 ……………… 75
13. 参考資料 ……………………… 78
    Emami の表 …………………… 78
    QUANTEC の表 ……………… 79
    小児耐容線量表 ………………… 81
    頭頸部のリンパ節領域 ………… 82
    頸部リンパ節転移の頻度 ……… 83
    医学生が知っておくべき
        放射線治療の知識 …………… 83
    医師国家試験出題基準に取り上げ
        られているキーワードの解説 … 84
    医学総論 ………………………… 84
    医学各論 ………………………… 89
    放射線治療の将来 ……………… 91
14. 略語 …………………………… 93

マニュアル改訂にあたって

　本書は、放射線治療ポケットマニュアルの4年後の改訂版である。改訂作業といえども、新しいマニュアルを作成するのと同等のエネルギーを要し、現在の放射線治療の進歩の速さには驚かされる。多くの知識は入れ替わる。知識の半減期は部門によって異なるが、年を追うごとに短くなり、積分値より微分係数が大事な時代になったと実感した。大改訂したために、本書のタイトルは"新"放射線治療ポケットマニュアルに変更した。

マニュアル作成にあたって

　本マニュアルは、日常の臨床に利用しやすいように、現在の標準治療をコンパクトに纏めたものである。常時、携帯し、折にふれて参照しやすいように、白衣の胸ポケットに入れられるサイズとした。東京医科大学では、新宿、茨城、八王子の3病院が同じガイドラインに沿って治療し、共通のデータベースで患者データを管理し、3病院全体の治療成績として報告することを目標にしている。これを実現する方法は、3病院で標準治療の考えをすり合わせて標準治療を実践することであり、この結果としてすべての医療機関で使用できる標準的なガイドラインが完成したと考えている。臨床試験にエントリーされた症例、関連科との治療の整合性からこの治療法をアレンジした場合以外では、このガイドラインに沿って治療を行っている。また、治療計画時に常時参照したい耐容線量についてはEmamiらによる古典的な表とそれを3次元治療に対応できるようにアップデートしたMarksらによる表、小児の耐容線量を参考資料として掲載した。医学生用に纏めた事項は卒業試験、国家試験対策としても役立つだけでなく、初期研修を終えて放射線科で研修を始める医師にも知識の整理に役立ててもらえるものと考えている。

序　文

　乳房温存術後に放射線治療を行うことが、標準的治療であることに異を唱える人は少ないと思う。"私の経験上あるいは施設の経験上"では乳房温存術の有効性は証明されなかった。有効性の証明には先人の長い時間と労力が必要であり、放射線腫瘍医は、標準的治療が確立されるまでの証拠を熟慮した上で診療に従事し、新たな臨床的課題を発見し解決していかなければならない。この Evidence making は大学に勤務している医師に課されている義務であると思う。この理解を助けるために、Evidence based medicine の考えに基づき、東京医科大学放射線科で施行するガイドラインを作成した。推奨線量設定の根拠は、国際的に評価された臨床試験グループによる結果より設定した。臨床試験により有効性が示されなかった場合、対象群による照射方法、線量を標準的治療と捉え設定した。このガイドラインが一般臨床のみならず、臨床的課題を解決するための臨床試験の発展に役立ち、より良い医療が施行されることを期待した。

1. 中枢神経

1-1. 悪性神経膠腫

術後照射として残存腫瘍に対して放射線治療を施行する。EORTCとNCI-Canadaの臨床研究において、残存腫瘍に2から3cmのマージンを加えて60Gy/30回照射をテモゾロマイドと同時併用することにより、照射単独に比較して生存期間が延長することが報告された[1, 2]。これに加え、MGMTプロモーターにメチル化が生じている場合が良好な予後因子であると報告された[3]。また、テモゾロマイド併用放射線療法にベバシズマブを併用することにより無増悪生存期間は延長したが、有意な生存延長効果は示されなかった[4]。線量および分割回数に関しては、60Gy/30回、60Gy/20回、40Gy/15回での照射を比較した臨床研究があるが、60Gy/30回と60Gy/20回では生存期間に有意差はなかったが、40Gy/15回で生存期間は有意に短縮した[5]。

70歳以上の高齢者においては放射線治療単独により無治療に比較して生存率が延長した[6]。この試験では残存腫瘍に対して2cmのマージンをとり50.4Gy/28回で施行した。同様に34Gy/10回照射、テモゾロマイド単独が標準の60Gy/30回照射より優れた生存率がえられている[7]。

照射野の設定
拡大局所：T2高信号＋1cmマージン
局所：Gd濃染領域＋1cmマージン

推奨線量
60Gy/30回（拡大局所40Gy、局所20Gy、テモゾロマイド併用）
50.4Gy/28回、34Gy/10回（70歳以上、放射線治療単独）

1-2. 低悪性度神経膠腫

早期に放射線治療を施行した場合と、症状の進行後に放射線治療を施行した場合、早期に放射線治療を施行した場合の方が、無病生存期間が長かったものの生存率に関して

は有意差を認めていない[8]。照射線量に関して、45Gy/25回と59.4Gy/33回[9]ならびに50.4Gy/28回と64.8Gy/36回[10]を比較した臨床試験が在るが、いずれも生存率、無病生存率とも有意差を認めなかった。

照射野の設定
局所：Gd濃染領域＋1cmマージン、照射野の縮小は困難

推奨線量
50.4Gy/28回

1-3. 脳胚腫

放射線治療によって治せる腫瘍であり、治さなくてはいけない腫瘍である。近年、放射線量を減らす臨床研究が行われているが、化学療法単独では治癒を望むことはできず、放射線治療は必須である[11]。

照射野の設定
全脳室照射＋局所

推奨線量
40Gy/20回（全脳室24Gy/12回、局所16Gy/8回）

1-4. 髄芽腫

基本的に根治を目指して術後照射を行う。髄膜播種を起こす確率が高いことから、全脳全脊髄照射の適応である[12]。

照射野の設定
全脳全脊髄＋後頭蓋窩

推奨線量
54Gy/27回（全脳全脊髄に標準リスク群で23.4Gy/13回、高リスク群で36Gy/20回、後頭蓋窩にブーストして総線量54Gy/30回）

1-5. 良性脳腫瘍

良性腫瘍であっても、十分な切除ができないことが多く、放射線治療が活躍する場は広い。脳神経領域は1回線量が副作用の発生に効いてくる領域であるので、1回線量は低く設定するのが望ましい。

1-5-1. 聴神経鞘腫

50.4Gy/28回と46.8Gy/26回の後ろ向きに検討した結果、制御率は両者とも100%であったが、聴力温存率は有意に低線量群で高かったとの報告がある[13]。聴神経鞘腫では聴力の温存の観点から、通常分割放射線治療が望ましい。特に55歳以上、3cm以上の腫瘍でその差が顕著である[14]。

照射野の設定
局所

推奨線量
46.8Gy/26回

1-5-2. 下垂体腺腫

通常照射の長い経験があり、通常分割が標準治療である。標準分割定位放射線治療は通常照射より、側頭葉壊死等の副作用の軽減が期待できることから、優れた方法と思われる。

照射野の設定
局所

推奨線量
50Gy/25回

1-5-3. 髄膜腫

基本は手術であり、確実には取りきれなかった症例、再発症例、悪性髄膜腫に対しては術後照射が必要である[15]。

[照射野の設定]

局所(dual tailを照射野に入れない)[16]

[推奨線量]

良性：50Gy/25回
悪性：60Gy/30回

1-5-4. 頭蓋咽頭腫

良性であるが浸潤傾向があり、放射線治療の適応である。有害事象を減らすために標準分割定位放射線治療は優れた治療法である[17]。

[照射野の設定]

局所

[推奨線量]

54Gy/30回

1) Stupp R et al: Radiotherapy plus concomitant and adjuvant temozolomide for glioblastoma. N Engl J Med 352(10): 987-996, 2005
2) Stupp R et al: Effects of radiotherapy with concomitant and adjuvant temozolomide versus radiotherapy alone on survival in glioblastoma in a randomised phase III study: 5-year analysis of the EORTC-NCIC trial. Lancet Oncol 10(5): 459-466, 2009
3) Hegi ME et al: MGMT gene silencing and benefit from temozolomide in glioblastoma. N Engl J Med 352(10): 997-1003, 2005
4) Chinot OL et al: Bevacizumab plus Radiotherapy–Temozolomide for Newly Diagnosed Glioblastoma. N Engl J Med 370(8): 709-722, 2014
5) Azoulay M et al: Comparison of radiation regimens in the treatment of Glioblastoma multiforme: results from a single institution. Radiat Oncol 10(1): 106, 2015
6) Cairncross G et al: Phase III trial of chemotherapy plus radiotherapy compared with radiotherapy alone for pure and mixed anaplastic oligodendroglioma: Intergroup Radiation Therapy Oncology Group Trial 9402. J Clin Oncol 24(18): 2707-2714, 2006
7) Malmström A et al: Temozolomide versus standard 6-week radiotherapy versus hypofractionated radiotherapy in patients older than 60 years with glioblastoma: the Nordic randomised, phase 3 trial. Lancet Oncol 13(9): 916-926, 2012

8) van den Bent MJ et al: Long-term efficacy of early versus delayed radiotherapy for low-grade astrocytoma and oligodendroglioma in adults: the EORTC 22845 randomised trial. Lancet 366(9490): 985-990, 2005
9) Karim AB et al: A randomized trial on dose-response in radiation therapy of low-grade cerebral glioma: European Organization for Research and Treatment of Cancer (EORTC) Study 22844. Int J Radiat Oncol Biol Phys 36(3): 549-556, 1996
10) Shaw E et al: Prospective randomized trial of low- versus high-dose radiation therapy in adults with supratentorial low-grade glioma: initial report of a North Central Cancer Treatment Group/Radiation Therapy Oncology Group/Eastern Cooperative Oncology Group study. J Clin Oncol 20(9): 2267-2276, 2002
11) Jensen AW et al: Long-term follow-up of dose-adapted and reduced-field radiotherapy with or without chemotherapy for central nervous system germinoma. Int J Radiat Oncol Biol Phys 77(5): 1449-1456, 2010
12) Packer RJ et al: Phase III study of craniospinal radiation therapy followed by adjuvant chemotherapy for newly diagnosed average-risk medulloblastoma. J Clin Oncol 24(25): 4202-4208, 2006
13) Andrews DW et al: Toward dose optimization for fractionated stereotactic radiotherapy for acoustic neuromas: comparison of two dose cohorts. Int J Radiat Oncol Biol Phys 74(2): 419-426, 2009
14) Fong BM et al: Hearing preservation after LINAC radiosurgery and LINAC radiotherapy for vestibular schwannoma. J Clin Neurosci 19(8): 1065-1070, 2012
15) Modha A et al: Diagnosis and treatment of atypical and anaplastic meningiomas : A review. Neurosurgery 57(3): 538-550, 2005
16) Bulthuis VJ et al: Gamma Knife radiosurgery for intracranial meningiomas: Do we need to treat the dural tail? A single center retrospective analysis and an overview of the literature. Surgical Neurology International 5: s391-s395, 2014
17) Harrabi SB et al: Long term results after fractionated stereotactic radiotherapy (FSRT) in patients with craniopharyngioma: maximal tumor control with minimal side effects. Radiat Oncol 9: 203-209, 2014

2. 頭頸部

2-1. 眼・眼窩腫瘍

まれな腫瘍で標準的な治療法は確立していない。網膜の耐容線量である40Gy/20回を考慮して放射線治療計画を立てる。

眼球内リンパ腫：血液・リンパ腫の項を参照。

2-1-1. 脈絡膜転移

CTVは脈絡膜として、4～6MV X線で30Gy/10回から40Gy/20回を予後により選択する。可能なら水晶体を照射野から外す。視力の維持または回復の率は90%である[1, 2]。多発脳転移があれば全脳と脈絡膜を同時に治療する。

[照射野の設定]

片側：脳転移、対側の脈絡膜転移が出現したときに治療ができるように、非共通面照射を施行。
両側：水晶体をはずすように前方の照射ラインを合わせるようにして両側脈絡膜を対向二門。

[推奨線量]

30Gy/10回、40Gy/20回

2-1-2. 網膜芽細胞腫

小児の一般的な眼の悪性腫瘍で、放射線治療単独により高い局所制御率が得られるため[3]初期治療として施行されていたが、顔面骨の変形、二次発癌の問題[4]より、化学療法による腫瘍縮小を図った後、レーザー光凝固、小線源治療などの局所療法を行い、残存した場合や再発後に施行される[5]。CTVは眼球として、可能なら水晶体を照射野から外す。4～6MV X線で41.4Gy/23回

[照射野の設定]

脈絡膜転移に準じる

[推奨線量]

41.4Gy/23回

2-1-3. 脈絡膜悪性黒色腫

陽子線治療[6, 7]あるいは^{125}Iシードなどを埋め込んだ円盤状の小線源を眼球の後面に張り付けるプラーク治療[8]により視力の温存が図られるが、視力の温存が不要の場合は定位放射線治療も可能である[9]。日本では陽子線施設で眼球治療用のアプリケータを保持している施設がないため、放医研の重粒子線治療に紹介する[10]。

[照射野の設定]

視神経の線量を低減するように設定

[推奨線量]

50Gy/5回
48Gy/6回

2-2. 鼻腔・副鼻腔癌

過去40年間、手術、放射線治療と化学療法の併用により、治療成績が向上している[11]。手術、化学療法に40〜60Gy/20〜30回の照射により、T4腫瘍においても5年生存率が50%を超えている[12, 13]。また、選択的動注併用し70Gy/35回の照射により、手術を施行しなくても同等の生存率が報告され化学放射線療法も選択される[14]。後ろ向きの研究において、IMRTは3DCRTに比較し局所制御率が向上している[15]。T4腫瘍であっても、他の頭頸部癌と違い頸部リンパ節再発は10%と少ないため、予防照射は不要と考えられている[16]。

> 照射野の設定

鼻腔全体、上顎洞全体、篩骨洞全体

> 推奨線量

手術併用：60～70Gy/30～35回
化学放射線療法：70Gy/35回（40Gy後にブースト）

2-3. 口唇と口腔癌（舌を除く）

　頬粘膜、上顎／下顎歯肉と歯槽、硬口蓋、舌（前方2/3）、口腔底の亜区域に分類される。T1-2N0では照射単独の治療が考えられるが、多くの場合術後照射として施行される[17]。他の頭頸部腫瘍と同様、術後に断端陽性や節外浸潤を認めた場合は化学放射線治療を行うことで生存率の向上を認めている[18, 19]。最近、選択的同側リンパ節廓清が再発後の廓清に比較して、全生存率の向上を認めており[20]、放射線治療においても選択的照射が必要であると考える。口腔癌は頤下、顎下リンパ節（LevelⅠ）とLevelⅡ、Ⅲの領域に転移しやすく[21～23]、対側へのリンパ節転移が少ないことが知られている[22, 24]。N0でありT2以下あるいは正中に近接していなければ対側のリンパ節照射は控えることを考慮する[22]。

　54Gy/27回以上でも顎骨壊死が増加するとの報告あり、同部位への照射を可能な限り抑える[25]。4～6MV X線により70Gyまで原発巣へ照射する。シェルを作成する時には口蓋に照射しなくてもよいように、マウスピースを用い舌と口蓋との距離をとる[26]。

> 照射野の設定

T1, 2N0原発巣ならびに同側のLevelⅠ-Ⅲのリンパ節領域
T3、N1以上、正中を超える場合は両側のLevelⅠ-Ⅲのリンパ節領域に必要なリンパ節領域を追加

> **推奨線量**
> 根治：70Gy/35回
> 術前：60～66Gy/30～33回

2-4. 舌癌

舌癌は口腔領域癌の50%を占める。T1N0は、小線源治療の適応である[27]。日本では低線量率線源を保有している施設は少なく、東京医科大学も低線量率線源は保有していないため、経験がある施設に紹介する。T2N0は小線源治療または外科的切除が適応で、T3以上では外科的切除の適応である。切除例で断端や節外浸潤陽性の際には化学放射線治療を行う[18, 19]。LevelⅠ-Ⅲに加え、他の口腔癌と異なりⅣへの転移が多い[21, 28]。

> **照射野の設定**
> 切除例で断端陽性：初期の照射野は原発と同側のLevelⅠ-Ⅳ、ブースト照射は原発部位。
> 節外浸潤：両側のLevelⅠ-Ⅴおよび腫瘍床、ブースト照射は節外部位。

> **推奨線量**
> 断端陽性例の術後照射：66Gy/33回
> 節外浸潤：60Gy/30回

2-5. 上咽頭癌

Ⅰ期は放射線単独[29]、Ⅱ期以上では化学放射線療法が行われる[30, 31]。5年生存率はⅡ期で80%[31]、Ⅲ期であっても70%を超える[32]良好な成績である。Ⅲ期でIMRTにより唾液分泌障害を軽減できたと報告されているが[33]、限局的である可能性がある[34]。当院ではSIB(Simultaneous integrated boost)法によるIMRTを行い、high risk PTV、intermidiate risk PTV、low risk PTVを設定している[35]。耳下腺への照射線量は平均で25Gyまでとする[36]。重篤な有害事象として、carotid blowout syndromeの報告されており過線量にならな

いように注意する[37]。

[照射野の設定]

IMRT：high risk 原発巣と有意なリンパ節、intermidiate risk 病側の頸部リンパ節領域、low risk 健側の頸部リンパ節領域、両側鎖骨上リンパ節領域

[推奨線量]

IMRT：high risk 70Gy/35回、intermediate risk 63Gy/35回、low risk 56Gy/35回

2-6. 中咽頭癌

舌根、喉頭蓋谷、扁桃、口蓋帆、後壁、軟口蓋に分けられる。病期Ⅰ-Ⅱ期は手術が、Ⅲ期に対して放射線治療を施行されることが多い。放射線治療単独に比較して化学療法を追加することにより、生存率の延長が報告されてから、化学放射線療法が一般的となっている[38,39]。切除可能なⅢ期例では切除±術後照射も行われるが、機能温存に優れた放射線治療が中心である[40]。Cetuximab併用放射線治療により、放射線単独に比較して局所制御率と生存率を向上させる[41]が、化学放射線療法への上乗せ効果は証明されていない[42]。従来はシスプラチンが用いられていたが、ドセタキセルを併用することにより生存率が向上している[43~45]が、毒性が強いことが問題である。

扁桃は対側へのリンパ節転移が少なく、舌根では両側リンパ節に転移しやすい。扁桃T1-2, N0であれば同側のLevel Ib-Vへ、T3-4, N0であれば両側のLevel Ib-Vへ、N+であればルビエールリンパ節を含める。舌根であればNにかかわらず、両側のLevel Ib-Vとルビエールリンパ節を照射範囲とする。軟口蓋で正中を超える場合はルビエールリンパ節を照射する[46]。原発巣を含め上記のリンパ節領域に対して44Gy/22回施行後に、原発巣と転移リンパ節に70Gy/35回照射する。HPV（またはp16）陽性で予後がよい[47]。

照射野の設定

原発巣、有意なリンパ節と予防リンパ節領域、ブースト照射は原発巣と有意なリンパ節

推奨線量

根治照射：70Gy/35回
術後照射：断端陽性66Gy/33回、その他60Gy/30回

2-7. 下咽頭癌

梨状陥凹、輪状後、後壁に分けられる。喉頭（発声機能）温存のため梨状陥凹原発の病期Ⅰ-Ⅱ期に対して化学放射線治療が選択さていた[48]が、病期Ⅲ期以上にも喉頭温存のみならず生存率の観点から推奨される[49]。原発巣のみが制御された場合、後に頸部郭清術を追加する選択肢もある。

梨状陥凹のN0は両側のLevel Ⅱ-Ⅳリンパ節領域[50, 51]を、後壁はLevel Ⅴとルビエールリンパ節を含める[46, 52]。N+の場合はさらにLevel Ⅴ-Ⅵ[53]と鎖骨上を含める。4～6MV X線で左右対向2門を基本に44Gy/22回照射後、70Gy/35回、原発巣および有意なリンパ節へブースト照射する。

照射野の設定

原発巣、有意なリンパ節と予防リンパ節領域、ブースト照射は原発巣と有意なリンパ節

推奨線量

根治照射：70Gy/35回
術後照射：断端陽性66Gy/33回、その他60Gy/30回

2-8. 喉頭癌

声門癌、声門上癌、声門下癌に分けられ、T1-2N0M0は放射線治療単独療法の適応である。病期Ⅲ-Ⅳ期以上はかつて手術適応であったが、多くの臨床試験の結果、2/3の患者において喉頭温存が達成されていることから化学放射線療法を勧めるべきである[54]。化学療法後に放射線治療を施行するより、同時に施行した方が、喉頭温存ならびに局所

制御率が優れていた[55]。

声門癌では、リンパ節転移はまれなため、局所照射のみを照射する。T3以上N+の場合は、Level Ⅱ-Ⅳを含める[46]。推奨総線量は、T1で66Gy/33回、T2以上で70Gy/35回である。

声門上ではN0の場合でもリンパ節転移が20%程度認め、両側のLevel Ⅱ-Ⅲを照射野に含む[56]。N+の場合はさらにLevel Ⅳ-Ⅴを含める[57]。Level Ⅱbへの転移が少ないため照射を控える[56, 57]。声門下ではⅡ-Ⅵを照射野[58]に含んで44Gy/22回照射の後、脊髄を外して局所ならびに有意なリンパ節へ照射する。推奨総線量は、T1で66Gy/33回、T2以上で70Gy/35回である。

| 照射野の設定 |

声門癌は、局所照射。声門上癌および声門下癌は、初期照射は頸部リンパ節領域を照射野に含む、ブースト照射は局所。

| 推奨線量 |

T1：66Gy/33回
T2以上：70Gy/35回
術後照射：断端陽性66Gy/33回、その他60Gy/30回

2-9. 耳下腺癌

外科的切除が第1選択である。比較試験はないが、1)腺様嚢胞癌などの高悪性度の場合、2)切除断端近接または陽性、3) T3-4、4)骨浸潤、5)神経周囲浸潤、6)リンパ節転移には、術後照射の有用性がみられた[59, 60]。切除不能例や再発例では放医研の重粒子線治療に紹介してもよい[61]。術後照射では、腫瘍床と同側Level Ⅰ-Ⅲ（低悪性度のN0は腫瘍床のみ）をCTVとして照射野を設定する[62]。腺様嚢胞癌では傍神経浸潤するため顔面神経に沿って頭蓋底まで照射する[63]。斜入2門wedge pairによる照射または3D-CRTやIMRTによって、総線量は、60Gy/30回。切除不能や再発例では70Gy/35回[59]まで行う。

照射野の設定

術後照射:腫瘍床と同側LevelⅠ-Ⅲ(低悪性度のN0は腫瘍床のみ)

注:腺様嚢胞癌では傍神経浸潤するため、腫瘍床は顔面神経にそって頭蓋底までである。

推奨線量

術後照射:60Gy/30回
切除不能や再発例:70Gy/35回

2-10. 甲状腺癌

分化型癌では、外科的切除が第1選択である。45歳以上で甲状腺外浸潤のあるもの(T4a, T4b)、顕微的腫瘍残存の疑われるときに推奨される[64]。切除不能や肉眼的残存では70Gy/35回まで照射する[65]。

未分化癌は、進行が急速で予後不良である。手術可能であれば術後に化学放射線療法を行う[66]。照射野や線量に定型的なものはなく、当院では局所と近接するリンパ節を含んで、急速な進行に対応するため1回1.5Gy、10回/週の加速多分割照射で60Gy/40回を施行する[67]。

照射野の設定

局所と近接するリンパ節

推奨線量

分化癌の切除不能や再発例:70Gy/35回
未分化癌:60Gy/40回(b.i.d)

2-11. 原発不明の頸部リンパ節転移

病理組織学的に扁平上皮癌か未分化癌である場合には、頭頸部癌が原発巣であるとして放射線療法を行うことに意義があるとされ、EBV, HPV/p16を参考にして上中咽頭癌に準じた化学放射線療法を行う[68, 69]。全頸部照射(LevelⅡ-Ⅴ、Ⅶ)とし、44Gy/22回以降は、腫大リンパ節に70Gy/35回、切除後であれば同部に60Gy/30回の照射とし

上中咽頭粘膜に66Gy/33回を照射する。

照射野の設定

初期の照射野は全頸部照射、ブースト照射は上中咽頭と有意なリンパ節

推奨線量

上中咽頭癌に準じる

1) Rudoler SB et al: External beam irradiation for choroid metastases: identification of factors predisposing to long-term sequelae. Int J Radiat Oncol Biol Phys 38(2): 251-256, 1997
2) Wiegel T et al: External beam radiotherapy of choroidal metastases−final results of a prospective study of the German Cancer Society (ARO 95-08). Radiother Oncol 64(1): 13-18, 2002
3) Singh AD et al: Relationship of regression pattern to recurrence in retinoblastoma. Br J Ophthalmol 77(1): 12-16, 1993
4) Kleinerman RA et al: Risk of new cancers after radiotherapy in long-term survivors of retinoblastoma: an extended follow-up. J Clin Oncol 23(10): 2272-2279, 2005
5) Shields CL et al: Chemoreduction plus focal therapy for retinoblastoma: factors predictive of need for treatment with external beam radiotherapy or enucleation. Am J Ophthalmol 133(5): 657-664, 2002
6) Gragoudas ES et al: Proton beam irradiation. An alternative to enucleation for intraocular melanomas. Ophthalmology 87(6): 571-581, 1980
7) Damato B et al: Proton beam radiotherapy of choroidal melanoma: the Liverpool-Clatterbridge experience. Int J Radiat Oncol Biol Phys 62(5): 1405-1411, 2005
8) Collaborative Ocular Melanoma Study G: The COMS randomized trial of iodine 125 brachytherapy for choroidal melanoma: V. Twelve-year mortality rates and prognostic factors: COMS report No. 28. Arch Ophthalmol 124(12): 1684-1693, 2006
9) Dunavoelgyi R et al: Hypofractionated stereotactic photon radiotherapy of posteriorly located choroidal melanoma with five fractions at ten Gy--clinical results after six years of experience. Radiother Oncol 108(2): 342-347, 2013
10) Tsuji H et al: Carbon-ion radiotherapy for locally advanced or unfavorably located choroidal melanoma: a Phase I / II dose-escalation study. Int J Radiat Oncol Biol Phys 67(3): 857-862, 2007
11) Dulguerov P et al: Nasal and paranasal sinus carcinoma: are we making progress? A series of 220 patients and a systematic review. Cancer 92(12): 3012-3029, 2001

12) Nibu K et al: Results of multimodality therapy for squamous cell carcinoma of maxillary sinus. Cancer 94(5): 1476-1482, 2002
13) Yoshimura R et al: Trimodal combination therapy for maxillary sinus carcinoma. Int J Radiat Oncol Biol Phys 53(3): 656-663, 2002
14) Homma A et al: Superselective high-dose cisplatin infusion with concomitant radiotherapy in patients with advanced cancer of the nasal cavity and paranasal sinuses: a single institution experience. Cancer 115(20): 4705-4714, 2009
15) Suh YG et al: Treatment outcomes of intensity-modulated radiotherapy versus 3D conformal radiotherapy for patients with maxillary sinus cancer in the postoperative setting. Head Neck, 2014
16) Homma A et al: Lymph node metastasis in t4 maxillary sinus squamous cell carcinoma: incidence and treatment outcome. Ann Surg Oncol 21(5): 1706-1710, 2014
17) Harrison LB et al: Radiation therapy for oral cavity cancer. Dent Clin North Am 34(2): 205-222, 1990
18) Bernier J et al: Postoperative irradiation with or without concomitant chemotherapy for locally advanced head and neck cancer. N Engl J Med 350(19): 1945-1952, 2004
19) Cooper JS et al: Postoperative concurrent radiotherapy and chemotherapy for high-risk squamous-cell carcinoma of the head and neck. N Engl J Med 350(19): 1937-1944, 2004
20) D'Cruz AK et al: Elective versus Therapeutic Neck Dissection in Node-Negative Oral Cancer. N Engl J Med 373(6): 521-529, 2015
21) Ferlito A et al: Elective management of the neck in oral cavity squamous carcinoma: current concepts supported by prospective studies. Br J Oral Maxillofac Surg 47(1): 5-9, 2009
22) Koo BS et al: Management of contralateral N0 neck in oral cavity squamous cell carcinoma. Head Neck 28(10): 896-901, 2006
23) Montes DM et al: Oral maxillary squamous carcinoma: an indication for neck dissection in the clinically negative neck. Head Neck 33(11): 1581-1585, 2011
24) Woolgar JA: Histological distribution of cervical lymph node metastases from intraoral/oropharyngeal squamous cell carcinomas. Br J Oral Maxillofac Surg 37(3): 175-180, 1999
25) Lee IJ et al: Risk factors and dose-effect relationship for mandibular osteoradionecrosis in oral and oropharyngeal cancer patients. Int J Radiat Oncol Biol Phys 75(4): 1084-1091, 2009
26) Kaanders JH et al: Devices valuable in head and neck radiotherapy. Int J Radiat Oncol Biol Phys 23(3): 639-645, 1992
27) Inoue T et al: Phase III trial of high- vs. low-dose-rate interstitial radiotherapy for early mobile tongue cancer. Int J Radiat Oncol Biol Phys 51(1): 171-175, 2001
28) Byers RM et al: Frequency and therapeutic implications of "skip me-

tastases" in the neck from squamous carcinoma of the oral tongue. Head Neck 19(1): 14-19, 1997
29) Cheng SH et al: Concomitant radiotherapy and chemotherapy for early-stage nasopharyngeal carcinoma. J Clin Oncol 18(10): 2040-2045, 2000
30) Baujat B et al: Chemotherapy in locally advanced nasopharyngeal carcinoma: an individual patient data meta-analysis of eight randomized trials and 1753 patients. Int J Radiat Oncol Biol Phys 64(1): 47-56, 2006
31) Chen QY et al: Concurrent chemoradiotherapy vs radiotherapy alone in stage Ⅱ nasopharyngeal carcinoma: phase Ⅲ randomized trial. J Natl Cancer Inst 103(23): 1761-1770, 2011
32) Wee J et al: Randomized trial of radiotherapy versus concurrent chemoradiotherapy followed by adjuvant chemotherapy in patients with American Joint Committee on Cancer/International Union against cancer stage Ⅲ and Ⅳ nasopharyngeal cancer of the endemic variety. J Clin Oncol 23(27): 6730-6738, 2005
33) Fang FM et al: Quality of life and survival outcome for patients with nasopharyngeal carcinoma receiving three-dimensional conformal radiotherapy vs. intensity-modulated radiotherapy-a longitudinal study. Int J Radiat Oncol Biol Phys 72(2): 356-364, 2008
34) Pow EH et al: Can intensity-modulated radiotherapy preserve oral health-related quality of life of nasopharyngeal carcinoma patients? Int J Radiat Oncol Biol Phys 83(2): e213-221, 2012
35) Lee N et al: Intensity-modulated radiation therapy with or without chemotherapy for nasopharyngeal carcinoma: radiation therapy oncology group phase Ⅱ trial 0225. J Clin Oncol 27(22): 3684-3690, 2009
36) Li Y et al: The impact of dose on parotid salivary recovery in head and neck cancer patients treated with radiation therapy. Int J Radiat Oncol Biol Phys 67(3): 660-669, 2007
37) Luo CB et al: Radiation carotid blowout syndrome in nasopharyngeal carcinoma: angiographic features and endovascular management. Otolaryngol Head Neck Surg 138(1): 86-91, 2008
38) Calais G et al: Randomized trial of radiation therapy versus concomitant chemotherapy and radiation therapy for advanced-stage oropharynx carcinoma. J Natl Cancer Inst 91(24): 2081-2086, 1999
39) Pignon JP et al: Meta-analysis of chemotherapy in head and neck cancer (MACH-NC): an update on 93 randomised trials and 17,346 patients. Radiother Oncol 92(1): 4-14, 2009
40) Soo KC et al: Surgery and adjuvant radiotherapy vs concurrent chemoradiotherapy in stage Ⅲ/Ⅳ nonmetastatic squamous cell head and neck cancer: a randomised comparison. Br J Cancer 93(3): 279-86, 2005
41) Bonner JA et al: Radiotherapy plus cetuximab for squamous-cell carci-

noma of the head and neck. N Engl J Med 354(6): 567-578, 2006
42) Ang KK et al: Randomized phase III trial of concurrent accelerated radiation plus cisplatin with or without cetuximab for stage III to IV head and neck carcinoma: RTOG 0522. J Clin Oncol 32(27): 2940-2950, 2014
43) Posner MR et al: Cisplatin and fluorouracil alone or with docetaxel in head and neck cancer. N Engl J Med 357(17): 1705-1715, 2007
44) Vermorken JB et al: Cisplatin, fluorouracil, and docetaxel in unresectable head and neck cancer. N Engl J Med 357(17): 1695-1704, 2007
45) Lorch JH et al: Induction chemotherapy with cisplatin and fluorouracil alone or in combination with docetaxel in locally advanced squamous-cell cancer of the head and neck: long-term results of the TAX 324 randomised phase 3 trial. Lancet Oncol 12(2): 153-159, 2011
46) Chao KS et al: Determination and delineation of nodal target volumes for head-and-neck cancer based on patterns of failure in patients receiving definitive and postoperative IMRT. Int J Radiat Oncol Biol Phys 53(5): 1174-1184, 2002
47) Ang KK et al: Human papillomavirus and survival of patients with oropharyngeal cancer. N Engl J Med 363(1): 24-35, 2010
48) Nakamura K et al: Chemoradiation therapy with or without salvage surgery for early squamous cell carcinoma of the hypopharynx. Int J Radiat Oncol Biol Phys 62(3): 680-683, 2005
49) Lefebvre JL et al: Phase 3 randomized trial on larynx preservation comparing sequential vs alternating chemotherapy and radiotherapy. J Natl Cancer Inst 101(3): 142-152, 2009
50) Buckley JG et al: Cervical node metastases in laryngeal and hypopharyngeal cancer: a prospective analysis of prevalence and distribution. Head Neck 22(4): 380-385, 2000
51) Koo BS et al: Management of contralateral N0 neck in pyriform sinus carcinoma. Laryngoscope 116(7): 1268-1272, 2006
52) Wu Z et al: Analysis of risk factors for retropharyngeal lymph node metastasis in carcinoma of the hypopharynx. Head Neck 35(9): 1274-1277, 2013
53) Joo YH et al: The impact of paratracheal lymph node metastasis in squamous cell carcinoma of the hypopharynx. Eur Arch Otorhinolaryngol 267(6): 945-950, 2010
54) Denaro N et al: A systematic review of current and emerging approaches in the field of larynx preservation. Radiother Oncol 110(1): 16-24, 2014
55) Forastiere AA et al: Concurrent chemotherapy and radiotherapy for organ preservation in advanced laryngeal cancer. N Engl J Med 349(22): 2091-2098, 2003
56) Jia S et al: Incidence of level IIB lymph node metastasis in supraglottic laryngeal squamous cell carcinoma with clinically negative neck–a

prospective study. Head Neck 35(7): 987-991, 2013
57) Lim YC et al: Level IIb lymph node metastasis in laryngeal squamous cell carcinoma. Laryngoscope 116(2): 268-272, 2006
58) Vorwerk H et al: Guidelines for delineation of lymphatic clinical target volumes for high conformal radiotherapy: head and neck region. Radiat Oncol 6: 97, 2011
59) Terhaard CH et al: The role of radiotherapy in the treatment of malignant salivary gland tumors. Int J Radiat Oncol Biol Phys 61(1): 103-111, 2005
60) Armstrong JG et al: Malignant tumors of major salivary gland origin. A matched-pair analysis of the role of combined surgery and postoperative radiotherapy. Arch Otolaryngol Head Neck Surg 116(3): 290-293, 1990
61) Schulz-Ertner D et al: Therapy strategies for locally advanced adenoid cystic carcinomas using modern radiation therapy techniques. Cancer 104(2): 338-344, 2005
62) Chen AM et al: Patterns of nodal relapse after surgery and postoperative radiation therapy for carcinomas of the major and minor salivary glands: what is the role of elective neck irradiation? Int J Radiat Oncol Biol Phys 67(4): 988-994, 2007
63) Gomez DR et al: Outcomes and prognostic variables in adenoid cystic carcinoma of the head and neck: a recent experience. Int J Radiat Oncol Biol Phys 70(5): 1365-1372, 2008
64) American Thyroid Association Guidelines Taskforce on Thyroid N, Differentiated Thyroid C, Cooper DS et al: Revised American Thyroid Association management guidelines for patients with thyroid nodules and differentiated thyroid cancer. Thyroid 19(11): 1167-1214, 2009
65) Rosenbluth BD et al: Intensity-modulated radiation therapy for the treatment of nonanaplastic thyroid cancer. Int J Radiat Oncol Biol Phys 63(5): 1419-1426, 2005
66) Kebebew E et al: Anaplastic thyroid carcinoma. Treatment outcome and prognostic factors. Cancer 103(7): 1330-1335, 2005
67) Wang Y et al: Clinical outcome of anaplastic thyroid carcinoma treated with radiotherapy of once- and twice-daily fractionation regimens. Cancer 107(8): 1786-1792, 2006
68) Strojan P et al: Contemporary management of lymph node metastases from an unknown primary to the neck: Ⅱ. a review of therapeutic options. Head Neck 35(2): 286-293, 2013
69) Wallace A et al: Head and neck squamous cell carcinoma from an unknown primary site. Am J Otolaryngol 32(4): 286-290, 2011

3. 胸部

3-1. 乳癌

乳房温存術後の放射線治療により乳房内再発率を抑制することを、多くの臨床試験の結果が示しているが[1-6]、メタ解析により10年後に4人の局所再発を抑制することにより15年後に1人の死亡を避けることが示された[7,8]。EORTCとカナダから照射領域に関して、鎖骨上、腋下と傍胸骨の所属リンパ節領域を含んで照射すると、乳腺のみの照射に比較して、局所再発と無病再発[9,10]あるいは乳癌死[10]を減少させると報告した。当院においては肺、心臓に対する線量を減少させるために、所属リンパ節に対してX線に電子線強度変調照射を併用している。

線量に関して、腫瘍床に対する追加照射により乳房内再発が減少することが示されていた[11-13]が、長期の経過観察において若年者ほどその効果が高い[12,14]。非浸潤性乳癌に対しても乳房温存術後の照射は推奨され[15-17]、追加照射の有効性も報告されている[18]。

乳房切除後に放射線治療を施行により生存率が改善し、再発率と乳癌死を低下させると報告され[19-21]、3個以上の転移のみならず[21]、1～3個のリンパ節転移においても、その有効性が確認された[20,22]。乳房温存術に準じて胸壁と所属リンパ節を含めて照射するが、年齢と分子生物学的な予後[23,24]を勘案して照射領域と線量を決定する。

照射野の設定

乳房温存術後：残存乳房、N1以上は鎖骨上窩、腋下、傍胸骨リンパ節を加える
乳房切除後：胸壁、N1以上は鎖骨上窩、腋下、傍胸骨リンパ節を加える

推奨線量

残存乳房または胸壁：50Gy/25回（断端陽性例では、局所に電子線で10Gy/5回を追加する）
鎖骨上窩、腋下、傍胸骨リンパ節領域：50Gy/25回（N1以上）

3-2. 非小細胞肺癌

●Ⅰ期

標準治療は手術であるが、優れた体幹部定位放射線治療の成績から、手術に代わる治療法として期待される。日本人の貢献が顕著な領域であり、本治療法により、約90％の局所制御が得られる[25~28]。至適線量は定まっていないが、本邦では48Gy/4回が最も多く用いられている[29]。手術可能な非小細胞肺癌に対して手術と体幹部定位放射線治療の2つの無作為比較試験が行われたが、予定数の症例集積ができずに終了となった（STARS, ROSEL）。この2つの試験58症例の統合解析の結果は、3年全生存率で手術群が79％、体幹部定位放射線治療群が95％で、後者においてハザード比が0.14に有意差をもって低下した[30]。しかし、本来の比較試験でないため、標準治療は依然として手術である。

照射野の設定

原発巣をCTVとする。呼吸移動分に1cmのマージンを設定。

推奨線量

48Gy/4回、75Gy/30回

●Ⅱ-Ⅲ期

1980年代にRTOGの報告で2年間の生存率において50Gyと60Gyでは後者の方が優れていたことより、60Gy/30回で照射することが非小細胞肺癌に対する標準的線量とされた[31]。それ以降、線量増加の有用性を検討する試験が数多く施行された[32]。しかし、RTOGにおける化学療法同時併用下での60Gyと74Gyの比較試験では、線量増加の有用性は認められなかったため、依然として60Gy/30回の照射が標準である[33]。Elective nodeの照射は不要である[34, 35]。照射野の決定にPETは有用であるので、治療前検査にPETを加えることが推奨される。

一方、Ⅳ期の治療において、EGFR遺伝子変異陽性例ではEGFR-TKIにより無病生存が改善し[36, 37]、ALK陽性例

にALK阻害剤の有効性が後ろ向き試験で示された[38]。放射線治療に併用する薬剤の今後の動向に注意を払う必要がある。

照射野の設定

原発巣＋有意なリンパ節（PETが有用）

推奨線量

60Gy/30回、66Gy/33回

3-3. 小細胞肺癌

限局型小細胞肺癌において、化学療法（cisplatinとetoposide）と同時併用して、総線量45Gyを1回1.5Gy、計30回を3週間で照射する1日2回照射法（BID）と1回1.8Gy、25回を5週間で照射する1日1回法を比較する第3相試験において、BIDにおいて2、5年生存率の向上[39]を認めた。現在、RTOG0538/CALGB30610において、標準とされている45Gy BID（1.5Gy/2回）、70Gy/35回（7週間）、61.2Gy/34回（16回を1日1回、残り18回をBID、計5週間）の第3相試験が進められている。

CRが得られた症例では、予防的全脳照射により限局型[40]、進展型[41]ともに生存率が延長し、進展型では胸部の放射線治療（30Gy/10回）により予後の延長が期待できる[42]。

照射野の設定

原発巣＋有意なリンパ節＋上縦隔リンパ節

推奨線量

45Gy（b.i.d）/30回
54.0Gy/30回
25Gy/10回（予防的全脳照射）

3-4. 胸腺腫・胸腺癌

MGHよりⅢ期の胸腺腫を対象に断端が近接していれば45から50Gy、顕微鏡的に断端陽性であれば54Gy、断端が

陽性であれば60Gy施行し、5年全生存率が71%と報告された[43]。Ⅱ期、Ⅲ期の治癒切除が成された場合の術後照射の有効性については証明されていない[44, 45]。

照射野の設定

原発巣、腫瘍床

推奨線量

60～70Gy（切除不能例）
50Gy/25回（顕微鏡的陽性）
60Gy/30回（肉眼的陽性）
治癒切除Ⅲ期
50Gy/25回

1) Clark RM et al: Randomized clinical trial of breast irradiation following lumpectomy and axillary dissection for node-negative breast cancer: an update. Ontario Clinical Oncology Group. J Natl Cancer Inst 88(22): 1659-1664, 1996
2) Fisher B et al: Twenty-year follow-up of a randomized trial comparing total mastectomy, lumpectomy, and lumpectomy plus irradiation for the treatment of invasive breast cancer. N Engl J Med 347(16): 1233-1241, 2002
3) Fisher B et al: Tamoxifen, radiation therapy, or both for prevention of ipsilateral breast tumor recurrence after lumpectomy in women with invasive breast cancers of one centimeter or less. J Clin Oncol 20(20): 4141-4149, 2002
4) Forrest AP et al: Randomised controlled trial of conservation therapy for breast cancer: 6-year analysis of the Scottish trial. Scottish Cancer Trials Breast Group. Lancet 348(9029): 708-713, 1996
5) Liljegren G et al: 10-Year results after sector resection with or without postoperative radiotherapy for stage I breast cancer: a randomized trial. J Clin Oncol 17(8): 2326-2333, 1999
6) Veronesi U et al: Radiotherapy after breast-preserving surgery in women with localized cancer of the breast. N Engl J Med 328(22): 1587-1591, 1993
7) Clarke M et al: Effects of radiotherapy and of differences in the extent of surgery for early breast cancer on local recurrence and 15-year survival: an overview of the randomised trials. Lancet 366(9503): 2087-2106, 2005

8) Early Breast Cancer Trialists' Collaborative G, Darby S et al: Effect of radiotherapy after breast-conserving surgery on 10-year recurrence and 15-year breast cancer death: meta-analysis of individual patient data for 10,801 women in 17 randomised trials. Lancet 378(9804): 1707-1716, 2011

9) Whelan TJ et al: Regional Nodal Irradiation in Early-Stage Breast Cancer. N Engl J Med 373(4): 307-316, 2015

10) Poortmans PM et al: Internal Mammary and Medial Supraclavicular Irradiation in Breast Cancer. N Engl J Med 373(4): 317-327, 2015

11) Bartelink H et al: Recurrence rates after treatment of breast cancer with standard radiotherapy with or without additional radiation. N Engl J Med 345(19): 1378-1387, 2001

12) Bartelink H et al: Impact of a higher radiation dose on local control and survival in breast-conserving therapy of early breast cancer: 10-year results of the randomized boost versus no boost EORTC 22881-10882 trial. J Clin Oncol 25(22): 3259-3265, 2007

13) Romestaing P et al: Role of a 10-Gy boost in the conservative treatment of early breast cancer: results of a randomized clinical trial in Lyon, France. J Clin Oncol 15(3): 963-968, 1997

14) Bartelink H et al: Whole-breast irradiation with or without a boost for patients treated with breast-conserving surgery for early breast cancer: 20-year follow-up of a randomised phase 3 trial. Lancet Oncol 16(1): 47-56, 2015

15) Fisher ER et al: Pathologic findings from the National Surgical Adjuvant Breast Project (NSABP) eight-year update of Protocol B-17: intraductal carcinoma. Cancer 86(3): 429-438, 1999

16) Houghton J et al: Radiotherapy and tamoxifen in women with completely excised ductal carcinoma in situ of the breast in the UK, Australia, and New Zealand: randomised controlled trial. Lancet 362(9378): 95-102, 2003

17) Julien JP et al: Radiotherapy in breast-conserving treatment for ductal carcinoma in situ: first results of the EORTC randomised phase III trial 10853. EORTC Breast Cancer Cooperative Group and EORTC Radiotherapy Group. Lancet 355(9203): 528-533, 2000

18) Omlin A et al: Boost radiotherapy in young women with ductal carcinoma in situ: a multicentre, retrospective study of the Rare Cancer Network. Lancet Oncol 7(8): 652-656, 2006

19) Overgaard M et al: Postoperative radiotherapy in high-risk premenopausal women with breast cancer who receive adjuvant chemotherapy. Danish Breast Cancer Cooperative Group 82b Trial. N Engl J Med 337(14): 949-955, 1997

20) Overgaard M et al: Postoperative radiotherapy in high-risk post-

menopausal breast-cancer patients given adjuvant tamoxifen: Danish Breast Cancer Cooperative Group DBCG 82c randomised trial. Lancet 353(9165): 1641-1648, 1999

21) Ragaz J et al: Adjuvant radiotherapy and chemotherapy in node-positive premenopausal women with breast cancer. N Engl J Med 337(14): 956-962, 1997

22) Ebctcg, McGale P et al: Effect of radiotherapy after mastectomy and axillary surgery on 10-year recurrence and 20-year breast cancer mortality: meta-analysis of individual patient data for 8135 women in 22 randomised trials. Lancet 383(9935): 2127-2135, 2014

23) Nguyen PL et al: Breast cancer subtype approximated by estrogen receptor, progesterone receptor, and HER-2 is associated with local and distant recurrence after breast-conserving therapy. J Clin Oncol 26(14): 2373-2378, 2008

24) Carey LA et al: Race, breast cancer subtypes, and survival in the Carolina Breast Cancer Study. JAMA 295(21): 2492-2502, 2006

25) Blomgren H et al: Stereotactic high dose fraction radiation therapy of extracranial tumors using an accelerator. Clinical experience of the first thirty-one patients. Acta Oncol 34(6): 861-870, 1995

26) Uematsu M et al: Computed tomography-guided frameless stereotactic radiotherapy for stage I non-small cell lung cancer: a 5-year experience. Int J Radiat Oncol Biol Phys 51(3): 666-670, 2001

27) Onishi H et al: Hypofractionated stereotactic radiotherapy (HypoFXSRT) for stage I non-small cell lung cancer: updated results of 257 patients in a Japanese multi-institutional study. J Thorac Oncol 2: S94-100, 2007

28) Timmerman R1 et al: Excessive toxicity when treating central tumors in a phase II study of stereotactic body radiation therapy for medically inoperable early-stage lung cancer. J Clin Oncol 24(30): 4833-4839, 2006

29) Nagata Y et al: Survey of stereotactic body radiation therapy in Japan by the Japan 3-D Conformal External Beam Radiotherapy Group. Int J Radiat Oncol Biol Phys 75(2): 343-347, 2009

30) Chang JY et al: Stereotactic ablative radiotherapy versus lobectomy for operable stage I non-small-cell lung cancer: a pooled analysis of two randomised trials. Lancet Oncol 16(6): 630-637, 2015

31) Perez CA et al: Patterns of tumor recurrence after definitive irradiation for inoperable non-oat cell carcinoma of the lung. Int J Radiat Oncol Biol Phys 6(8): 987-994, 1980

32) Bradley JD et al: A phase I/II radiation dose escalation study with concurrent chemotherapy for patients with inoperable stag-

es I to Ⅲ non-small-cell lung cancer: phase I results of RTOG 0117. Int J Radiat Oncol Biol Phys 77(2): 367-372, 2010
33) Bradley JD et al: Standard-dose versus high-dose conformal radiotherapy with concurrent and consolidation carboplatin plus paclitaxel with or without cetuximab for patients with stage ⅢA or ⅢB non-small-cell lung cancer (RTOG 0617): a randomised, two-by-two factorial phase 3 study. Lancet Oncol 16(2): 187-199, 2015
34) Schild SE et al: Results of a Phase I Trial of Concurrent Chemotherapy and Escalating Doses of Radiation for Unresectable Non-Small Cell Lung Cancer. Int J Radiat Oncol Biol Phys 65(4): 1106-1111, 2006
35) Socinski MA et al: Randomized phase Ⅱ trial of induction chemotherapy followed by concurrent chemotherapy and dose-escalated thoracic conformal radiotherapy (74Gy) in stage III non-small-cell lung cancer: CALGB 30105. J Clin Oncol 26(15): 2457-2463, 2008
36) Maemondo M et al: Gefitinib or chemotherapy for non-small-cell lung cancer with mutated EGFR. N Engl J Med 362(25): 2380-2388, 2010
37) Inoue A et al: Updated overall survival results from a randomized phase Ⅲ trial comparing gefitinib with carboplatin-paclitaxel for chemo-naïve non-small cell lung cancer with sensitive EGFR gene mutations (NEJ002). Ann Oncol 24(1): 54-59, 2013
38) Shaw AT et al: Effect of crizotinib on overall survival in patients with advanced non-small-cell lung cancer harbouring ALK gene rearrangement: a retrospective analysis. Lancet Oncol 12(11): 1004-1012, 2011
39) Turrisi AT 3rd et al: Twice-daily compared with once-daily thoracic radiotherapy in limited small-cell lung cancer treated concurrently with cisplatin and etoposide. N Engl J Med 340(4): 265-271, 1999
40) Auperin A et al: Prophylactic cranial irradiation for patients with small-cell lung cancer in complete remission. Prophylactic Cranial Irradiation Overview Collaborative Group. N Engl J Med 341(7): 476-484, 1999
41) Slotman B et al: Prophylactic cranial irradiation in extensive small-cell lung cancer. N Engl J Med 357(7): 664-672, 2007
42) Slotman BJ et al: Use of thoracic radiotherapy for extensive stage small-cell lung cancer: a phase 3 randomised controlled trial. Lancet 385(9962): 36-42, 2015
43) Myojin M et al: Stage Ⅲ thymoma: pattern of failure after surgery and postoperative radiotherapy and its implication for future study. Int J Radiat Oncol Biol Phys 46(4): 927-933, 2000
44) Chen YD et al: Role of adjuvant radiotherapy for stage Ⅱ thymoma after complete tumor resection. Int J Radiat Oncol Biol Phys

45) Ogawa K et al: Postoperative radiotherapy for patients with completely resected thymoma: a multi-institutional, retrospective review of 103 patients. Cancer 94(5): 1405-1413, 2002

memo

4. 消化器

4-1. 食道癌

　JCOG9907により術後化学療法に比較して術前化学療法により生存率が優れていた[1]ことから、日本においてはT4腫瘍を除く病期Ⅱ-Ⅲ期の食道癌において、術前化学療法後の手術が標準的と考えられている。MRCでは術前化学療法が手術単独治療に比較して生存率が優れていた[2]が、RTOGにおいては証明されていない[3,4]。一方、欧米では術前化学放射線療法が手術単独に比較して優れた生存率が報告され[5-8]、また、術前化学療法よりも化学放射線療法による生存率の向上[9]が報告されている。

　RTOG85-01では64Gy/32回の放射線治療単独と50.4Gy/28回の化学放射線療法が比較され[10,11]、化学放射線療法の有効性が示された。最近のメタ解析においても化学放射線療法の有効性が示されている[12]。至適線量に関して、INT0123において線量増加による生存率、局所制御率の向上を認めなかった[13]ため、CDDP+5FU併用50.4Gy/28回が標準と考えられる。しかし日本では、INT0123への批判と、JCOG9906の照射線量[14]から根治照射として60Gy/30回により化学放射線療法が施行されることが多い[15]。病期Ⅰ期に対しては日本から手術と同等な優れた生存率が報告されており[16-18]、積極的に化学放射線療法を勧めるべきである。

　化学放射線療法は局所再発を50%[5,10,13]に認めるために、手術が可能な場合は術前照射を考慮する。2つの化学放射線療法単独と術前化学放射線治療後に手術を施行する比較試験が施行され、両者の比劣勢が証明されている。治療関連死は手術併用に、局所再発は化学放射線療法に多かった[19,20]。化学放射線療法後の局所再発はQOLを低下させるため、手術が安全に施行される場合は手術を施行すべきと考える。照射線量は欧米においては40～50Gy施行される[6,8,21]が、当院においては30Gy/15回の術前照射により70%に病期を低下させ良好な成績を得ている[22]。

　照射範囲に関して、外科切除の報告を参照すると予防リ

ンパ節への照射が妥当と考えられ[23]、鎖骨上窩、傍食道、縦隔、噴門部周囲リンパ節領域を含み、上部食道に主座がある場合は頸部リンパ節を、下部食道の場合は腹腔動脈リンパ節領域をさらに含める[24]。ブーストは腫瘍の頭尾方向3cm[25]と有意なリンパ節を含める。

照射野の設定

鎖骨窩から噴門部(上部食道は頸部リンパ節、下部食道癌は腹腔動脈リンパ節を含める)。ブーストは原発巣と有意なリンパ節。

推奨線量

根治的化学放射線療法:61.2Gy/34回(41.4Gy/23回後はブースト)

術前化学放射線療法:30Gy/15回、40回Gy/20回

4-2. 結腸癌

放射線治療を推奨するRCTはない[26]。術後照射に関する有用性の報告があるが臨床試験で行う[27-29]。

4-3. 直腸癌

1980年代の直腸癌の術後に化学放射線療法により局所制御率が向上するとの結果[30-32]より、1990年にNIHが病期Ⅱ、Ⅲ期の直腸癌に対して術後化学放射線療法を標準的治療として推奨した[33]。1997年にスウェーデンより術前に25Gy/5回で照射すると手術単独に比較して、局所制御率のみならず生存率が向上したとの結果が得られた[34]。オランダにおいても25Gy/5回術前に施行により、局所制御率は有意差を認めたが、生存率では認めなかった[35, 36]。ドイツにおいてT3、T4あるいはリンパ節陽性を対象に、5FUを併用した50.4Gy/28回の術前照射と術後照射を比較した結果、術前照射の方が局所制御率と直腸の温存率が高く、有害事象発生率が低かった[37]ことより、術前照射が標準的治療と考えられるようになった。抗癌剤の有効性は証明され

ていないが[38~40]、5FUにオキサリプラチンの併用により無病生存率の延長を認めている[41]。25Gy/5回の短期照射も同等と考えられるが、遠位直腸に対する通常照射の有効性から[42]50.4Gyにより施行している。手術単独に比べ、晩期の小腸閉塞、肛門括約筋機能低下が多い[43, 44]。照射領域は45Gyまで直腸周囲、仙骨前面、内腸骨動脈領域[45]、下部総腸骨動脈領域[46]を照射し、5.4Gyを腫瘍に対してブーストしている。

照射野の設定
直腸周囲、仙骨前面、内腸骨動脈領域45Gy照射後、腫瘍の周囲に対して5.4Gyのブーストを施行。

推奨線量
直腸癌:50.4Gy/28回

4-4. 肛門管癌

術前に5FUとMMC併用の化学放射線治療を行うと高い腫瘍反応を得たことから[47]、放射線治療単独と5FU/MMC併用の化学放射線治療を比較し、化学放射線療法により局所制御と肛門温存の向上を認めた[48~50]。放射線治療に5FU単剤は5FU/MMCに比較して局所制御率、生存率、肛門温存率が劣る[51]。5FU/CDDPと5FU/MMCの比較試験は、RTOGにおいて45～59.4Gy/25～33回併用により、5FU/MMCが肛門温存率、無病生存率[52]、生存率が優れ[53]、英国から50.4Gy/28回により有意性を示せなかった[54]ため、5FU/MMC併用放射線治療が標準的である。両者の差はMMCの投与量、照射線量がRTOGの方が多いことにあるかもしれない。

照射野の設定
T1N0:会陰部皮膚を含む肛門管から、仙腸関節の下端。外腸骨、閉鎖リンパ節、後側は仙骨前面、鼠径リンパ節に照射。

肺経リンパ節は36Gy/20回で終了。
T2以上あるいはN+：上記より総腸骨動脈下端まで含める。
45Gy/25回後、腫瘍のみに縮小し59.4Gyまで施行する。
肺経リンパ節は電子線で照射し、N0であれば36Gy/20回で終了、N1であれば54Gy/30回まで施行[52]。

推奨線量

T1N0：50.4Gy/28回
T2以上あるいはN+：59.4Gy/33回

4-5. 原発性肝癌

肝癌ガイドラインでは、放射線治療の有効性において高いレベルのエビデンスはないとされており、門脈腫瘍栓症例や切除不能症例、内科的合併症などの理由で、他の標準的な治療法が適応とならない病態に対しては、3次元原体照射法による放射線治療を検討してよいとされている。陽子線治療の研究成果[55〜57]からは、Child-Pughスコアが10点以下で、全く照射されない正常肝を500mL以上確保できれば陽子線治療は可能であると考えられ、このデータを基に放射線治療の適応を考えることができる。門脈腫瘍栓（PVTT）[58]や右葉か左葉に限局した肝細胞癌（安全に照射できれば皮膜外浸潤やサテライトがあってもよい）が主な適応となる。また、下大静脈腫瘍栓に対しても適応となる[59]。

処方線量として、60Gyを20〜30回分割（1回2〜3Gy）して照射することによりgrade3以上の有害事象がみられなかった[60, 61]。照射法は、多門照射やノンコプラナーを用いて耐容線量以上が照射される肝臓の容積を減らすように局在に応じて工夫する。また、定位放射線治療は将来性のある治療法であるが、最適な照射体積の設定方法、線量分割方法は定まっていない。

照射野の設定

造影CTで認められる腫瘍から5mmのマージンをとってCTVとする。

> **推奨線量**
> 危険臓器が近接しない場合：60Gy/30回
> 危険臓器が近接する場合：50.4Gy/28Fr回

4-6. 胆管癌

根治治療としては切除術が第1選択である。胆嚢癌に対して大規模なランダム化比較試験は行われておらず、放射線療法の意義は十分に確立されているとはいえない。放射線療法は切除不能例や術後の断端陽性例、リンパ節転移を有する症例に関しては術後照射の適応となる[62]。また、除痛・減黄・ステント開存期間延長を目的とした対症療法としての放射線治療を施行する場合も多い。

処方線量として、腸管を完全に避けられるようであれば60Gy/30回、避けられない場合は50.4Gy/28回の照射を行う。照射範囲として、肝内胆管癌の切除片解析ではGTVに5〜8mmのマージンを加えてCTVとすることが推奨されている[63]。

> **照射野の設定**
> 術後照射：腫瘍床および陽性リンパ節に対して5mmほどのマージンを加えてCTVとする。
> 切除不能症例：GTV（陽性リンパ節を含める）に5〜10mm程度のマージンを加えてCTVとする。

> **推奨線量**
> 危険臓器が近接しない場合：60Gy/30回
> 危険臓器が近接する場合：50.4Gy/28回

4-7. 膵癌

膵癌は難治癌の代表であり、切除可能例は20％前後で、その5年生存率は20％程度である。およそ半数は遠隔転移例で長期予後は望み難い。残り30〜40％の切除不能局所進行例が化学放射線療法の適応となる。また、術前の補助療法としての照射や、癌疼痛に対する緩和的照射も行われる。

膵癌診療ガイドラインでは局所進行切除不能膵癌に対する一次治療として、化学放線療法または化学療法単独による治療を推奨している。ECOGでは局所進行切除不能膵癌に対してゲムシタビン塩酸塩併用での放射線療法（50.4Gy/28Fr）群とゲムシタビン塩酸塩による化学療法単独群とに割り付けるランダム化比較試験を実施しており、化学放射線療法群の生存期間が有意に良好であったと報告している[64]。また、2006年に膵癌に対して保険適応となったS-1と放射線療法との併用についての報告があり[65, 66]、これらの放射線療法のレジメンも50Gy程度の線量が用いられている。局所進行切除不能癌の治療成績は、ゲムシタビン塩酸塩やS-1などの抗癌剤薬を用いた治療により少しずつ向上してきている。

　照射範囲に関しては、膵癌は原発巣自体の制御が困難であり、予防的リンパ節領域まで照射野に含める意義は乏しいとする考え方がある。GTV＋転移頻度の高いリンパ節群をCTVとして照射を行い、治療はほとんどの症例で完遂可能で、照射野外リンパ節再発はなかったという報告がある[67, 68]。また、照射技術的にはSBRTやIMRTで線量の集中性を高める方法も用いられるようになってきたが、照射範囲の比較については今後の臨床試験による検証が必要と考えられる。

照射野の設定

腫瘍のある部位とリンパ節のある部位、および腹腔動脈幹より上腸管膜動脈までの後腹膜をCTVとする。

推奨線量

50.4Gy/28回（非切除、不完全治癒切除、術前）

1) Ando N et al: A randomized trial comparing postoperative adjuvant chemotherapy with cisplatin and 5-fluorouracil versus preoperative chemotherapy for localized advanced squamous cell carcinoma of the thoracic esophagus (JCOG9907). Ann Surg Oncol 19(1): 68-74, 2012
2) Cunningham D et al: Perioperative chemotherapy versus surgery

alone for resectable gastroesophageal cancer. N Engl J Med 355(1): 11-20, 2006
3) Kelsen DP et al: Chemotherapy followed by surgery compared with surgery alone for localized esophageal cancer. N Engl J Med 339(27): 1979-1984, 1998
4) Kelsen DP et al: Long-term results of RTOG trial 8911 (USA Intergroup 113): a random assignment trial comparison of chemotherapy followed by surgery compared with surgery alone for esophageal cancer. J Clin Oncol 25(24): 3719-3725, 2007
5) Oppedijk V et al: Patterns of recurrence after surgery alone versus preoperative chemoradiotherapy and surgery in the CROSS trials. J Clin Oncol 32(5): 385-391, 2014
6) Tepper J et al: Phase III trial of trimodality therapy with cisplatin, fluorouracil, radiotherapy, and surgery compared with surgery alone for esophageal cancer: CALGB 9781. J Clin Oncol 26(7): 1086-1092, 2008
7) Shapiro J et al: Neoadjuvant chemoradiotherapy plus surgery versus surgery alone for oesophageal or junctional cancer (CROSS): long-term results of a randomised controlled trial. Lancet Oncol 16(9): 1090-1098, 2015
8) van Hagen P et al: Preoperative chemoradiotherapy for esophageal or junctional cancer. N Engl J Med 366(22): 2074-2084, 2012
9) Gebski V et al: Survival benefits from neoadjuvant chemoradiotherapy or chemotherapy in oesophageal carcinoma: a meta-analysis. Lancet Oncol 8(3): 226-234, 2007
10) Cooper JS et al: Chemoradiotherapy of locally advanced esophageal cancer: long-term follow-up of a prospective randomized trial (RTOG 85-01). Radiation Therapy Oncology Group. JAMA 281(17): 1623-1627, 1999
11) Herskovic A et al: Combined chemotherapy and radiotherapy compared with radiotherapy alone in patients with cancer of the esophagus. N Engl J Med 326(24): 1593-1598, 1992
12) Zhu LL et al: A Meta-Analysis of Concurrent Chemoradiotherapy for Advanced Esophageal Cancer. PLoS One 10:e0128616, 2015
13) Minsky BD et al: INT 0123 (Radiation Therapy Oncology Group 94-05) phase III trial of combined-modality therapy for esophageal cancer: high-dose versus standard-dose radiation therapy. J Clin Oncol 20(5): 1167-1174, 2002
14) Ohtsu A et al: Definitive chemoradiotherapy for T4 and/or M1 lymph node squamous cell carcinoma of the esophagus. J Clin Oncol 17(9): 2915-2921, 1999
15) Nishimura Y et al: Clinical outcomes of radiotherapy for esophageal cancer between 2004 and 2008: the second survey of the Japanese Radiation Oncology Study Group (JROSG). Int J Clin On-

col, 2015
16) Kato H et al: A phase II trial of chemoradiotherapy for stage I esophageal squamous cell carcinoma: Japan Clinical Oncology Group Study (JCOG9708). Jpn J Clin Oncol 39(10):638-643, 2009
17) Sai H et al: Long-term results of definitive radiotherapy for stage I esophageal cancer. Int J Radiat Oncol Biol Phys 62(5): 1339-1344, 2005
18) Yamada K et al: Treatment results of chemoradiotherapy for clinical stage I (T1N0M0) esophageal carcinoma. Int J Radiat Oncol Biol Phys 64(4): 1106-1111, 2006
19) Bedenne L et al: Chemoradiation followed by surgery compared with chemoradiation alone in squamous cancer of the esophagus: FFCD 9102. J Clin Oncol 25(10): 1160-1168, 2007
20) Stahl M et al: Chemoradiation with and without surgery in patients with locally advanced squamous cell carcinoma of the esophagus. J Clin Oncol 23(10): 2310-2317, 2005
21) Urba SG et al: Randomized trial of preoperative chemoradiation versus surgery alone in patients with locoregional esophageal carcinoma. J Clin Oncol 19(2): 305-313, 2001
22) Kobayashi N et al: Tumor response after low-dose preoperative radiotherapy combined with chemotherapy for squamous cell esophageal carcinoma. Anticancer Res 33(3): 1157-1161, 2013
23) Akiyama H et al: Radical lymph node dissection for cancer of the thoracic esophagus. Ann Surg 220(3): 364-72; discussion 372-373, 1994
24) Onozawa M et al: Elective nodal irradiation (ENI) in definitive chemoradiotherapy (CRT) for squamous cell carcinoma of the thoracic esophagus. Radiother Oncol 92(2): 266-269, 2009
25) Gao XS et al: Pathological analysis of clinical target volume margin for radiotherapy in patients with esophageal and gastroesophageal junction carcinoma. Int J Radiat Oncol Biol Phys 67(2): 389-396, 2007
26) Martenson JA et al: Phase III study of adjuvant chemotherapy and radiation therapy compared with chemotherapy alone in the surgical adjuvant treatment of colon cancer: results of intergroup protocol 0130. J Clin Oncol 22(16): 3277-3283, 2004
27) Amos EH et al: Postoperative radiotherapy for locally advanced colon cancer. Ann Surg Oncol 3(5): 431-436, 1996
28) Gunderson LL et al: Locally advanced primary colorectal cancer: intraoperative electron and external beam irradiation +/- 5-FU. Int J Radiat Oncol Biol Phys 37(3): 601-614, 1997
29) Willett CG et al: Does postoperative irradiation play a role in the adjuvant therapy of stage T4 colon cancer? Cancer J Sci Am 5(4): 242-247, 1999

30) Fisher B et al: Postoperative adjuvant chemotherapy or radiation therapy for rectal cancer: results from NSABP protocol R-01. J Natl Cancer Inst 80(1): 21-29, 1988
31) Krook JE et al: Effective surgical adjuvant therapy for high-risk rectal carcinoma. N Engl J Med 324(11): 709-715, 1991
32) Thomas PR et al: Adjuvant postoperative radiotherapy and chemotherapy in rectal carcinoma: a review of the Gastrointestinal Tumor Study Group experience. Radiother Oncol 13(4): 245-252, 1988
33) NIH consensus conference. Adjuvant therapy for patients with colon and rectal cancer. JAMA 264(11): 1444-1450, 1990
34) Improved survival with preoperative radiotherapy in resectable rectal cancer. Swedish Rectal Cancer Trial. N Engl J Med 336(14): 980-987, 1997
35) Kapiteijn E et al: Preoperative radiotherapy combined with total mesorectal excision for resectable rectal cancer. N Engl J Med 345(9): 638-646, 2001
36) Peeters KC et al: The TME trial after a median follow-up of 6 years: increased local control but no survival benefit in irradiated patients with resectable rectal carcinoma. Ann Surg 246(5): 693-701, 2007
37) Sauer R et al: Preoperative versus postoperative chemoradiotherapy for rectal cancer. N Engl J Med 351(17): 1731-1740, 2004
38) Gerard JP et al: Preoperative radiotherapy with or without concurrent fluorouracil and leucovorin in T3-4 rectal cancers: results of FFCD 9203. J Clin Oncol 24(28): 4620-4625, 2006
39) Bosset JF et al: Fluorouracil-based adjuvant chemotherapy after preoperative chemoradiotherapy in rectal cancer: long-term results of the EORTC 22921 randomised study. Lancet Oncol 15(2): 184-190, 2014
40) Breugom AJ et al: Adjuvant chemotherapy after preoperative (chemo)radiotherapy and surgery for patients with rectal cancer: a systematic review and meta-analysis of individual patient data. Lancet Oncol 16(2): 200-2007, 2015
41) Rodel C et al: Oxaliplatin added to fluorouracil-based preoperative chemoradiotherapy and postoperative chemotherapy of locally advanced rectal cancer (the German CAO/ARO/AIO-04 study): final results of the multicentre, open-label, randomised, phase 3 trial. Lancet Oncol 16(8): 979-989, 2015
42) Ngan SY et al: Randomized trial of short-course radiotherapy versus long-course chemoradiation comparing rates of local recurrence in patients with T3 rectal cancer: Trans-Tasman Radiation Oncology Group trial 01.04. J Clin Oncol 30(31): 3827-3833, 2012
43) Birgisson H et al: Late gastrointestinal disorders after rectal can-

44) Pollack J et al: Long-term effect of preoperative radiation therapy on anorectal function. Dis Colon Rectum 49(3): 345-352, 2006
45) Myerson RJ et al: Elective clinical target volumes for conformal therapy in anorectal cancer: a radiation therapy oncology group consensus panel contouring atlas. Int J Radiat Oncol Biol Phys 74(3): 824-830, 2009
46) Samuelian JM et al: Reduced acute bowel toxicity in patients treated with intensity-modulated radiotherapy for rectal cancer. Int J Radiat Oncol Biol Phys 82(5): 1981-1987, 2012
47) Leichman L et al: Cancer of the anal canal. Model for preoperative adjuvant combined modality therapy. Am J Med 78(1): 211-215, 1985
48) Epidermoid anal cancer: results from the UKCCCR randomised trial of radiotherapy alone versus radiotherapy, 5-fluorouracil, and mitomycin. UKCCCR Anal Cancer Trial Working Party. UK Co-ordinating Committee on Cancer Research. Lancet 348(9034): 1049-1054, 1996
49) Bartelink H et al: Concomitant radiotherapy and chemotherapy is superior to radiotherapy alone in the treatment of locally advanced anal cancer: results of a phase III randomized trial of the European Organization for Research and Treatment of Cancer Radiotherapy and Gastrointestinal Cooperative Groups. J Clin Oncol 15(5): 2040-2049, 1997
50) Northover J et al: Chemoradiation for the treatment of epidermoid anal cancer: 13-year follow-up of the first randomised UKCCCR Anal Cancer Trial (ACT I). Br J Cancer 102(7): 1123-1128, 2010
51) Flam M et al: Role of mitomycin in combination with fluorouracil and radiotherapy, and of salvage chemoradiation in the definitive nonsurgical treatment of epidermoid carcinoma of the anal canal: results of a phase III randomized intergroup study. J Clin Oncol 14(9): 2527-2539, 1996
52) Ajani JA et al: Fluorouracil, mitomycin, and radiotherapy vs fluorouracil, cisplatin, and radiotherapy for treatment of the anal canal: a randomized controlled trial. JAMA 299(16): 1914-1921, 2008
53) Gunderson LL et al: Long-term update of US GI intergroup RTOG 98-11 phase III trial for anal carcinoma: survival, relapse, and colostomy failure with concurrent chemoradiation involving fluorouracil/mitomycin versus fluorouracil/cisplatin. J Clin Oncol 30(35): 4344-4351, 2012
54) James RD et al: Mitomycin or cisplatin chemoradiation with or without maintenance chemotherapy for treatment of squamous-cell carcinoma of the anus (ACT II): a randomised, phase 3, open-

label, 2 x 2 factorial trial. Lancet Oncol 14(6): 516-524, 2013
55) Chiba T et al: Proton beam therapy for hepatocellular carcinoma: a retrospective review of 162 patients. Clin Cancer Res 11(10): 3799-3805, 2005
56) Nakayama H et al: Proton beam therapy for hepatocellular carcinoma: the University of Tsukuba experience. Cancer 115(23): 5499-5506, 2009
57) Hashimoto T et al: Repeated proton beam therapy for hepatocellular carcinoma. Int J Radiat Oncol Biol Phys 65(1): 196-202, 2006
58) Sugahara S et al: Proton-beam therapy for hepatocellular carcinoma associated with portal vein tumor thrombosis. Strahlenther Onkol 185(12): 782-788, 2009
59) Mizumoto M et al: Proton beam therapy for hepatocellular carcinoma with inferior vena cava tumor thrombus: report of three cases. Jpn J Clin Oncol 37(6): 459-462, 2007
60) Huang Y et al: The treatment responses in cases of radiation therapy to portal vein thrombosis in advanced hepatocellular carcinoma. Int J Radiat Oncol Biol Phys 73(4): 1155-1163, 2009
61) Zhang XB et al: Hepatocellular carcinoma with main portal vein tumor thrombus: treatment with 3-dimensional conformal radiotherapy after portal vein stenting and transarterial chemoembolization. Cancer 115(6): 1245-1252, 2009
62) National comprehensive cancer network NCCN Clinical Practice Guidelines in Oncology Hepatobiliary Cancers. 2012
63) Bi AH et al: Impact factors for microinvasion in intrahepatic cholangiocarcinoma: A possible system for defining clinical target volume. Int J Radiat Oncol Biol Phys 78(5): 1427-1436, 2010
64) Loehrer PJ Sr et al: Gemcitabine alone versus gemcitabine plus radiotherapy in patients with locally advanced pancreatic cancer: an Eastern Cooperative Oncology Group trial. J Clin Oncol 29(31): 4105-4112, 2011
65) Sudo K et al: Phase II study of oral S-1 and concurrent radiotherapy in patients with unresectable locally advanced pancreatic cancer. Int J Radiat Oncol Biol Phys 80(1):119-125, 2011
66) Ikeda M et al: A multicenter phase II trial of S-1 with concurrent radiation therapy for locally advanced pancreatic cancer. Int J Radiat Oncol Biol Phys 85(1): 163-169, 2013
67) Kawakami H et al: Toxicities and effects of involved-field irradiation with concurrent cisplatin for unresectable carcinoma of the pancreas. Int J Radiat Oncol Biol Phys 62(5): 1357-1362, 2005
68) Tokuuye K et al: Small-field radiotherapy in combination with concomitant chemotherapy for locally advanced pancreatic carcinoma. Radiother Oncol 67(3): 327-330, 2003

5. 泌尿器

5-1. 膀胱癌

浸潤性膀胱癌で膀胱温存を希望している手術拒否例や手術不能例が適応となる。陽子線治療の検討から膀胱の側壁および前壁は従来いわれている60Gy/30回よりも耐容は高いと考えられる[1]。根治的膀胱全摘除術との比較試験はなされていないものの、化学放射線療法は放射線治療単独と比べて局所制御を改善し[2]、手術療法に匹敵する高い治療成績が得られている。放射線治療の処方線量およびその方法については、40〜50Gyまで骨盤リンパ節領域を含め前後左右の4門で行い、その後に膀胱に限局して60〜70Gyまで治療を行うプロトコルが一般的である[3, 4]。RTOG89-03ではCDDPと併用により39.6Gy/22回施行後、膀胱鏡により完全寛解を得られた場合に、追加照射を施行し64.8Gy/36回まで施行し、CR率60％、2年膀胱温存率82％を得ている[5]。完全寛解に至らない場合は膀胱切除が施行された。よって39.6Gy/22回施行後に腸管が完全に避けられるようであれば、64.8Gy/36回、不可能な場合は50.4Gy/28回に留める。

照射野の設定

初期の照射野は膀胱全体と内腸骨動脈リンパ節を含む。ブースト照射は局所。

推奨線量

腸管が近接しない場合：64.8Gy/36回
腸管が近接する場合：50.4Gy/28回

5-2. 前立腺癌（外照射）

リスクグループ（低リスク（PSA＜10、GS＜7、T1-2aN0M0の3つを満たすもの）、高リスク（PSA＞20、GS＞7、T3aN0以上のいずれかを満たすもの）、中リスク（低リスクでも高リスクでもないもの））に分けて[6]、治療方法を決定する。低リスクは放射線治療単独。中リスクはホルモン療法（Maximal androgen block：MABを6ヵ月併用（3

～6ヵ月先行の後で放射線治療開始)。高リスクはホルモン療法を2年併用(3～6ヵ月先行の後で放射線治療開始)。PIVOT studyではPSA値が10以下、低リスクグループでは手術による致死率の低下は認められなかった。治療の適応の決定は慎重に行い、有害事象を出さない治療が重要である[7]。

全摘除術後の断端陽性例やPSA再発例も外照射の適応となる。ASTROコンセンサスパネルでは、64Gy以上の線量が推奨されている[8]。

[照射野の設定]

低リスクは前立腺全体、中リスクは精囊基部も含めて前立腺全体、高リスクは小骨盤をCTVとして開始。44Gy/22回で直腸側を中心にマージンを縮小し、直腸側のマージンは3～5mmとし膀胱側のマージンも5mm以下とする。60Gy/30回で精囊を外せる症例では外して直腸の線量分布によっては直腸側のマージンを3mm以下にしてもよい。多門照射や回転原体照射で行う場合は総線量74Gy/37回[9]まで施行。Field in Field法を用いて直腸の線量を落としてもよい。

IMRTで行う場合は、直腸のV70が5%以下になるような計画を目指す。初期の照射野は精囊基部も含めて前立腺全体をCTVとする。40Gy後は直腸側のマージンを縮小、60Gy後は精囊を外す。

[推奨線量]

74Gy/37回、IMRTで行う場合は、さらに線量を増加する(78Gy/39回)
全摘除術後(断端陽性例やPSA再発例):64Gy/32回

5-3. 精巣腫瘍

放射線治療の適応は、主にⅠ・Ⅱ期のセミノーマの術後照射である[10]。

Ⅰ期では、JonesらのRCTの結果、30Gy/15回と20Gy/10回で効果に差がなく、晩期障害は30Gy/15回の方が多いこ

とが明らかになっているため[11]、線量は21.6Gy/12回とする。また、照射野は傍大動脈リンパ節だけでもよいという説が有力である。

ⅡA期は、従来から用いられている患側の骨盤内リンパ節と傍大動脈リンパ節に対して30.6Gy/17回、ⅡB期は、36.0Gy/20回を処方線量とする。

> 照射野の設定

Ⅰ期：傍大動脈リンパ節
Ⅱ期：患側の骨盤内リンパ節と傍大動脈リンパ節

> 推奨線量

術後照射としてⅠ期：21.6Gy/12回
ⅡA期：30.6Gy/17回
ⅡB期：36.0Gy/20回

1) Hata M et al: Proton beam therapy for invasive bladder cancer: a prospective study of bladder-preserving therapy with combined radiotherapy and intra-arterial chemotherapy. Int J Radiat Oncol Biol Phys 64(5): 1371-1379, 2006
2) James ND et al: Radiotherapy with or without chemotherapy in muscle-invasive bladder cancer. N Engl J Med 366(16): 1477-1488, 2012
3) Rödel C et al: Trimodality treatment and selective organpreservation for bladder cancer. J Clin Oncol 24(35): 5536-5544, 2006
4) Pos FJ et al: Radical radiotherapy for invasive bladder cancer: What dose and fractionation schedule to choose? Int JRadiat Oncol Biol Phys 64(4): 1168-1173, 2006
5) Tester W et al: Neoadjuvant combined modality program with selective organ preservation for invasive bladder cancer: results of Radiation Therapy Oncology Group phase Ⅱ trial 8802. J Clin Oncol 14(1): 119-126, 1996
6) D'Amico AV et al: Predicting prostate specific antigen outcome preoperatively in the prostate specific antigen era. J Urol 166(6): 2185-2188, 2001
7) Wilt TJ et al: Radical prostatectomy versus observation for localized prostate cancer. N Engl J Med 367(3): 203-213, 2012
8) Cox JD et al: Consensus statements on radiation therapy of prostate cancer: guidelines for prostate re-biopsy after radiation and for radiation therapy with rising prostate-specific antigenlevels

9) Kupelian PA et al: Radical prostatectomy, external beam radiotherapy <72 Gy, external beam radiotherapy $>$ or $=72$ Gy, permanent seed implantation, or combined seeds/external beam radiotherapy for stage T1-T2 prostate cancer. Int J Radiat Oncol Biol Phys 58(1): 25-33, 2004
10) Schmoll HJ et al: European consensus on diagnosis and treatment of germ cell cancer: a report of the European Germ Cell Cancer Consensus Group (EGCCCG). Ann Oncol 15(9): 1377-1399, 2004
11) Jones WG et al: Randomized trial of 30 versus 20 Gy in the adjuvant treatment of stage I Testicular Seminoma: a report on Medical Research Council Trial TE18, European Organisation for the Research and Treatment of Cancer Trial 30942 (ISRCTN18525328). J Clin Oncol 23(6): 1200-1208, 2005

(Note: The list continues from a previous page; item 8 ends at "1155, 1999" at the top: "after radical prostatectomy. American Society for Therapeutic Radiology and Oncology Consensus Panel. J Clin Oncol 17(4): 1155, 1999")

6. 婦人科癌

6-1. 子宮頸癌

RTOG90-01により放射線単独と比べてシスプラチン、5FU併用放射線治療による生存率の延長が報告された[1, 2]。GOGからはシスプラチン、5FU併用放射線療法がヒドロキシウレア併用放射線治療に比較して[3]、またシスプラチン、シスプラチンと5FUとヒドロキシウレア、ヒドロキシウレアと放射線療法の比較においてシスプラチン併用放射線治療による生存率の向上を認めた[4]。これらの結果から、日本においてもシスプラチンに外照射50.4Gy/28回の骨盤照射(19.8〜41.4Gyで中央遮蔽)が施行される。それに加えて腔内照射A点線量6Gyで2〜4回投与する。IMRTを用いる場合は、中央遮蔽は使用せず、50.4Gy/28回の照射後に腔内照射A点線量6Gyを2〜3回追加する。IMRT使用により消化管有害事象の低減につながる[5]。ガーゼ(および綿球)のパッキングを十分に行って子宮と直腸間の距離できるだけ離して直腸線量を減らす。東京医大においては、アプリケータ挿入下でMRIあるいはCTによる画像誘導小線源治療を行い、腫瘍に対する線量の評価[6]と直腸線量を低下させている[7]。

術後化学放射線治療により生存率の向上が報告されている[8〜12]。リンパ節転移陽性[9, 11]、断端陽性[12〜14]、高度な筋層浸潤[8〜10, 13, 15, 16]、子宮傍結合組織浸潤[9, 10, 13]、リンパ管侵襲[8〜10, 13, 15〜17]、腺癌あるいは腺扁平上皮癌[9, 10]を認める場合は、45Gy/25回の全骨盤照射に、局所照射を追加し50.4Gy/28回(リンパ節の局在によっては傍大動脈リンパ節へ延長)を行う。膣断端陽性例については、45Gy/25回の後に膣腔内照射を1回5Gyで2回追加する。

照射野の設定

初期の照射は全骨盤
ブースト照射は腔内照射

> [推奨線量]

根治照射：50.4Gy/28回の骨盤照射（19.8～41.4Gyで中央遮蔽または中央遮蔽なし）＋腔内照射A点線量6Gy×2～4回。

IMRTを用いる場合：50.4Gy/28回の骨盤照射（中央遮蔽なし）＋腔内照射A点線量6Gy×2～3回。

術後照射：45Gy/25回の骨盤照射±5.4Gy/3回の局所照射、膣断端陽性なら膣用のアプリケータで5Gy×2回追加。

6-2. 子宮体癌

子宮体癌の85％は切除可能な早期癌とされ、手術が第一選択となる。術後照射においても低－中リスクにおいては生存率の向上を認めず[18～20]、また20年以後の二次発癌増加の結果もでており注意が必要である[20, 21]。外照射に代わり、腔内照射の有効性が報告されている[22]。膣断端陽性なら膣用のアプリケータで粘膜下5mmに6Gyの腔内照射を2～3回追加する。

手術非適応例の体癌では、放射線治療が行われるが、骨盤照射50.4Gyに40Gy程度で中央遮蔽を行い、腔内照射を6Gy×2～3回追加する。

> [照射野の設定]

初期の照射は全骨盤
ブースト照射は腔内照射

> [推奨線量]

術後照射：50.4Gy/28回。膣断端陽性なら膣用のアプリケータで6Gy×2回追加。

根治照射：50.4Gy/28回の全骨盤照射（39.6Gyで中央遮蔽）＋腔内照射6Gy×2～3回

6-3. 膣・外陰癌

　膣癌では、いずれの病期においても放射線治療が選択肢としてあげられる。FIGO Ⅱ期でもリンパ節転移の頻度が25〜30%あるので、表在癌を除いては、全骨盤照射45〜50Gyを先行し[23]、さらに膣用のアプリケータで粘膜下5mmで5〜7Gy、アプリケータ表面線量が8〜12Gyの腔内照射を3〜4回追加する。膣の下1/3は鼠径リンパ節が所属リンパ節なので、電子線で鼠径部の予防照射45〜50Gyも追加する。

　外陰癌は手術が選択される場合も多く、術前、術後や再発時に放射線治療が選択される。化学放射線治療についても臨床研究が重ねられているが、現時点で手術に優る結果は示されていない[24]。浅く限局している場合（概ね4cm以下）は、局所へ電子線を用いて60〜70Gy/30〜35回の照射を行う。根治を狙う場合はcN0でも鼠径部の予防照射45〜50Gyも追加する。鼠径リンパ節が陽性例に根治照射を行う時は、全骨盤＋鼠径リンパ節＋外陰にX線照射を先行する。電子線治療は砕石位での照射になる。外陰の粘膜炎はかなり強くなるので50Gy程度でうまく外尿道孔などが外せれば鉛ブロックなどで遮蔽する。膣方向（深部方向）への進展が深い場合は膣癌に準じて治療する。

照射野の設定

　膣癌：初期の照射野は全骨盤（膣の下1/3は鼠径リンパ節も含む）。ブースト照射は腔内照射。
　外陰癌：局所＋鼠径リンパ節（上記も参照）

推奨線量

　膣癌：45〜50Gy＋膣用のアプリケータで5〜7Gy×3〜4回追加。
　外陰癌：60〜70Gy/30〜35回

1) Eifel PJ et al: Pelvic irradiation with concurrent chemotherapy versus pelvic and para-aortic irradiation for high-risk cervical

cancer: an update of radiation therapy oncology group trial (RTOG)90-01. J Clin Oncol 22(5): 872-880, 2004
2) Morris M et al: Pelvic radiation with concurrent chemotherapy compared with pelvic and para-aortic radiation for high-risk cervical cancer. N Engl J Med 340(15): 1137-1143, 1999
3) Whitney CW et al: Randomized comparison of fluorouracil plus cisplatin versus hydroxyurea as an adjunct to radiation therapy in stage ⅡB-ⅣA carcinoma of the cervix with negative para-aortic lymph nodes: a Gynecologic Oncology Group and Southwest Oncology Group study. J Clin Oncol 17(5): 1339-1348, 1999
4) Rose PG et al: Concurrent cisplatin-based radiotherapy and chemotherapy for locally advanced cervical cancer. N Engl J Med 340(14): 1144-1153, 1999
5) Gandhi AK et al: Early clinical outcomes and toxicity of intensity modulated versus conventional pelvic radiation therapy for locally advanced cervix carcinoma: a prospective randomized study. Int J Radiat Oncol Biol Phys 87(3): 542-548, 2013
6) Dimopoulos JC et al: Dose-volume histogram parameters and local tumor control in magnetic resonance image-guided cervical cancer brachytherapy. Int J Radiat Oncol Biol Phys 75(1): 56-63, 2009
7) Georg P et al: Dose-volume histogram parameters and late side effects in magnetic resonance image-guided adaptive cervical cancer brachytherapy. Int J Radiat Oncol Biol Phys 79(2): 356-362, 2011
8) Peters WA 3rd et al: Concurrent chemotherapy and pelvic radiation therapy compared with pelvic radiation therapy alone as adjuvant therapy after radical surgery in high-risk early-stage cancer of the cervix. J Clin Oncol 18(8): 1606-1613, 2000
9) Noh JM et al: Comparison of clinical outcomes of adenocarcinoma and adenosquamous carcinoma in uterine cervical cancer patients receiving surgical resection followed by radiotherapy: a multicenter retrospective study (KROG 13-10). Gynecol Oncol 132(3): 618-623, 2014
10) Ryu SY et al: Intermediate-risk grouping of cervical cancer patients treated with radical hysterectomy: a Korean Gynecologic Oncology Group study. Br J Cancer 110(2): 278-285, 2014
11) Monk BJ et al: Rethinking the use of radiation and chemotherapy after radical hysterectomy: a clinical-pathologic analysis of a Gynecologic Oncology Group/Southwest Oncology Group/Radiation Therapy Oncology Group trial. Gynecol Oncol 96(3): 721-728, 2005
12) Estape RE et al: Close vaginal margins as a prognostic factor after radical hysterectomy. Gynecol Oncol 68(3): 229-232, 1998

13) Chernofsky MR et al: Influence of quantity of lymph vascular space invasion on time to recurrence in women with early-stage squamous cancer of the cervix. Gynecol Oncol 100(2): 288-293, 2006
14) Diaz ES et al: Predictors of residual carcinoma or carcinoma-in-situ at hysterectomy following cervical conization with positive margins. Gynecol Oncol 132(1): 76-80, 2014
15) Rotman M et al: A phase III randomized trial of postoperative pelvic irradiation in Stage IB cervical carcinoma with poor prognostic features: follow-up of a gynecologic oncology group study. Int J Radiat Oncol Biol Phys 65(1): 169-176, 2006
16) Sedlis A et al: A randomized trial of pelvic radiation therapy versus no further therapy in selected patients with stage IB carcinoma of the cervix after radical hysterectomy and pelvic lymphadenectomy: A Gynecologic Oncology Group Study. Gynecol Oncol 73(2): 177-183, 1999
17) Marchiole P et al: Clinical significance of lympho vascular space involvement and lymph node micrometastases in early-stage cervical cancer: a retrospective case-control surgico-pathological study. Gynecol Oncol 97(3): 727-732, 2005
18) Creutzberg CL et al: Surgery and postoperative radiotherapy versus surgery alone for patients with stage-1 endometrial carcinoma: multicentre randomised trial. PORTEC Study Group. Post Operative Radiation Therapy in Endometrial Carcinoma. Lancet 355(9213): 1404-1411, 2000
19) Keys HM et al: A phase III trial of surgery with or without adjunctive external pelvic radiation therapy in intermediate risk endometrial adenocarcinoma: a Gynecologic Oncology Group study. Gynecol Oncol 92(3): 744-751, 2004
20) Onsrud M et al: Long-term outcomes after pelvic radiation for early-stage endometrial cancer. J Clin Oncol 31(31): 3951-3956, 2013
21) Chaturvedi AK et al: Second cancers among 104,760 survivors of cervical cancer: evaluation of long-term risk. J Natl Cancer Inst 99(21): 1634-1643, 2007
22) Nout RA et al: Vaginal brachytherapy versus pelvic external beam radiotherapy for patients with endometrial cancer of high-intermediate risk (PORTEC-2): an open-label, non-inferiority, randomised trial. Lancet 375(9717): 816-823, 2010
23) Frank SJ et al: Definitive radiation therapy for squamous cell carcinoma of the vagina. Int J Radiat Oncol Biol Phys 62(1): 138-147, 2005
24) Shylasree TS et al: Chemoradiation for advanced primary vulval cancer. Cochrane Database Syst Rev:CD003752, 2011

7. 血液・リンパ腫

7-1. 非ホジキンリンパ腫

濾胞性リンパ腫、病期Ⅰ-Ⅱ期の第一選択は放射線治療である[1~4]。大規模なデータベースからも放射線治療が他の治療に比較して無病生存率と生存率が高いことが示された[5, 6]。

びまん性大細胞型に関して、SWOGにおいてⅠ-Ⅱ期の中悪性度リンパ腫を対象に、CHOP 8コース施行とCHOP 3コース施行後に放射線治療を40～50Gy施行を比較したところ、5年生存率において放射線治療併用群の方が局所制御率、生存率とも良好であった[7]が、10年生存率には差を認めなかった。ECOGにおいてCHOP 8コース施行後に放射線治療30～40Gy施行したところ生存率に差を認めないものの照射施行の方が局所制御率は良好であった[8]。後ろ向きの研究ではリツキサンを併用するR-CHOPに放射線治療を併用することでR-CHOPのみに比較して、無病生存率と生存率の改善が報告されている[9~11]。Involved fieldとinvolved siteを照射する比較試験において両者に局所再発率と生存率の差を認めていない[12]。

胃悪性リンパ腫に対しては、ピロリ菌の除菌を施行後[13]、残存を認める場合に放射線治療を施行する[14, 15]。

照射野の設定

Involved siteをCTVとする。

推奨線量

Follicular lymphoma：30Gy/15回
Diffuse large B cell lymphoma：40Gy/20回、46Gy/23回（bulky）
・眼窩、結膜リンパ腫
  Follicular lymphoma：30Gy/15回
  Marginal zone B cell lymphoma：30Gy/15回
  Diffuse large B cell lymphoma：40Gy/20回

・胃悪性リンパ腫
　　Marginal zone B cell lymphoma：30Gy/15回
　　Diffuse large B cell lymphoma：40Gy/20回

7-2. ホジキンリンパ腫

　病期Ⅰ-Ⅱ期を対象とした、GHSG HD10ではABVDを4コースあるいは2コース後に、放射線治療を30Gy/15回あるいは20Gy/10回を組み合わせて4群の比較をおこなった。ABVD2コース後に20Gy/10回を施行した群が他の群と比較して非劣勢が証明された[16]。HD 11では予後不良群にABVDあるいはBEACOPP後に20Gyあるいは30Gy施行し、ABVD 4コース後に30Gyの照射が推奨された[17]。BEACOPPのABVDに対する有効性はECOGの試験でも示されていない[18]。involved fieldに照射、MOPPとABVを6コース施行後にinvolved fieldに照射、MOPPとABVを4コース施行後にsubtotal nodalに照射する比較試験を施行した。線量は36Gy/18回後、腫瘍の残存があれば4Gy/2回追加した。10年生存率で有意差を認めなかったことよりMOPPとABVを4コース施行後のinvolved field照射を標準的治療とすべきと結論付けた[19]。Ⅲ-Ⅳ期に対しても化学療法後の残存病変に放射線治療が考慮される[20]。Involved fieldが用いられていたが、involved node による照射の有効性が証明されている[21, 22]。

　予後のよいnodular lymphocyte predominant HD、病期Ⅰ-Ⅱ期に対しても放射線治療が第一選択となる[23]。

照射野の設定

Involved nodeをCTVとする。
予後良好群：ABVD 2あるいは4コース後にCRは20Gy/10回、PRは30Gy/15回
予後不良群：ABVD 4コース後に30Gy/15回

1) Guadagnolo BA et al: Long-term outcome and mortality trends in early-stage, Grade 1-2 follicular lymphoma treated with radiation

therapy. Int J Radiat Oncol Biol Phys. 64(3): 928-934, 2006
2) Mac Manus MP et al: Is radiotherapy curative for stage I and II low-grade follicular lymphoma? Results of a long-term follow-up study of patients treated at Stanford University. J Clin Oncol 14(4): 1282-1290, 1996
3) Vaughan Hudson B et al: Clinical stage 1 non-Hodgkin's lymphoma: long-term follow-up of patients treated by the British National Lymphoma Investigation with radiotherapy alone as initial therapy. British journal of cancer 69(6): 1088-1093, 1994
4) Wilder RB et al: Long-term results with radiotherapy for Stage I-II follicular lymphomas. Int J Radiat Oncol Biol Phys 51(5): 1219-1227, 2001
5) Pugh TJ et al: Improved survival in patients with early stage low-grade follicular lymphoma treated with radiation: a Surveillance, Epidemiology, and End Results database analysis. Cancer 116(16): 3843-3851, 2010
6) Vargo JA et al: What is the optimal management of early-stage low-grade follicular lymphoma in the modern era? Cancer 121(18): 2235-3334, 2015
7) Miller TP et al: Chemotherapy alone compared with chemotherapy plus radiotherapy for localized intermediate- and high-grade non-Hodgkin's lymphoma. N Engl J Med 339(1): 21-26, 1998
8) Horning SJ et al: Chemotherapy with or without radiotherapy in limited-stage diffuse aggressive non-Hodgkin's lymphoma: Eastern Cooperative Oncology Group study 1484. J Clin Oncol 22(15): 3032-3038, 2004
9) Marcheselli L et al: Radiation therapy improves treatment outcome in patients with diffuse large B-cell lymphoma. Leuk Lymphoma 52(10): 1867-1872, 2011
10) Kwon J et al: Additional survival benefit of involved-lesion radiation therapy after R-CHOP chemotherapy in limited stage diffuse large B-cell lymphoma. Int J Radiat Oncol Biol Phys 92(1): 91-98, 2015
11) Phan J et al: Benefit of consolidative radiation therapy in patients with diffuse large B-cell lymphoma treated with R-CHOP chemotherapy. J Clin Oncol 28(27): 4170-4176, 2010
12) Campbell BA et al: Limited-stage diffuse large B-cell lymphoma treated with abbreviated systemic therapy and consolidation radiotherapy: involved-field versus involved-node radiotherapy. Cancer 118(17): 4156-4165, 2012
13) Wotherspoon AC et al: Regression of primary low-grade B-cell gastric lymphoma of mucosa-associated lymphoid tissue type after eradication of Helicobacter pylori. Lancet 342(8871): 575-577, 1993

14) Schechter NR et al: Treatment of mucosa-associated lymphoid tissue lymphoma of the stomach with radiation alone. J Clin Oncol 16(5): 1916-1921, 1998
15) Tsang RW et al: Stage I and Ⅱ MALT lymphoma: results of treatment with radiotherapy. Int J Radiat Oncol Biol Phys. 50(5): 1258-1264, 2001
16) Engert A et al: Reduced treatment intensity in patients with early-stage Hodgkin's lymphoma. N Engl J Med 363(7): 640-652, 2010
17) Eich HT et al: Intensified chemotherapy and dose-reduced involved-field radiotherapy in patients with early unfavorable Hodgkin's lymphoma: final analysis of the German Hodgkin Study Group HD11 trial. J Clin Oncol 28(27): 4199-4206, 2010
18) Advani RH et al: Randomized Phase Ⅲ Trial Comparing ABVD Plus Radiotherapy With the Stanford V Regimen in Patients With Stages I or Ⅱ Locally Extensive, Bulky Mediastinal Hodgkin Lymphoma: A Subset Analysis of the North American Intergroup E2496 Trial. J Clin Oncol 33(17): 1936-1942, 2015
19) Ferme C et al: Chemotherapy plus involved-field radiation in early-stage Hodgkin's disease. N Engl J Med 357(19): 1916-1927, 2007
20) Engert A et al: Reduced-intensity chemotherapy and PET-guided radiotherapy in patients with advanced stage Hodgkin's lymphoma (HD15 trial): a randomised, open-label, phase 3 non-inferiority trial. Lancet 379(9828): 1791-1799, 2012
21) Campbell BA et al: Involved-nodal radiation therapy as a component of combination therapy for limited-stage Hodgkin's lymphoma: a question of field size. J Clin Oncol 26(32): 5170-5174, 2008
22) Paumier A et al: Involved-node radiotherapy and modern radiation treatment techniques in patients with Hodgkin lymphoma. Int J Radiat Oncol Biol Phys. 80(1): 199-205, 2011
23) Nogova L et al: Extended field radiotherapy, combined modality treatment or involved field radiotherapy for patients with stage IA lymphocyte-predominant Hodgkin's lymphoma: a retrospective analysis from the German Hodgkin Study Group (GHSG). Annals of oncology 16(10): 1683-1687, 2005

8. 緩和

8-1. 転移性脳腫瘍

転移性脳腫瘍の予後予測は治療法を適切に選択する上で重要であり、RTOGの臨床試験の結果を集約したRecursive partitioning analysis (RPA)[1]やGraded Prognostic Assessment (GPA)[2]が一般に用いられている。単発の転移性脳腫瘍を外科切除後に全脳照射を施行することにより、頭蓋内再発を抑制し、神経原性の死亡を減らすことが示されている[3]。

RTOGにおいて1から3個の転移性脳腫瘍に対して全脳照射37.5Gy/15回施行単独と定位放射線治療併用とを比較した結果、併用群においてRPA class IやGPA高値であれば生存率も向上することが示された[4,5]。投与線量はRTOG第I相試験の結果から、辺縁線量として24.0Gy/1回 (≤2cm)、18.0Gy/1回 (>2cm、≤3cm)、15.0Gy/1回 (>3cm、≤4cm) が推奨される[6]。JROSGにおいては1~4個の転移性脳腫瘍に対して定位放射線治療単独と全脳照射併用を比較した。初期の報告では、全脳照射併用により新たな脳転移の出現を抑制し、局所制御率を向上するが、生存期間の延長は認められないと結論づけたが[7]、その後の長期経過観察の報告では、予後良好群では全脳照射を併用することにより生存期間の延長が認められた[8]。学習、記憶能力についてSRS単独とSRSと全脳照射群との比較試験では4ヵ月後の計測において前者で有意に脳機能が保たれる一方、脳内の再発率は増加した。単独治療と頻回な経過観察を推奨している[9]。

[照射野の設定]

全脳または局所（上記参照）

[推奨線量]

5個以上の転移：全脳照射30Gy/10回（全身状態不良の場合

は20Gy/5回も考慮される)
2から4個の転移：全脳照射30Gy/10回±定位照射
1個の転移：定位照射（線量は本文参照）

注1：定位照射において1回で照射を行う場合はstereotactic radiosurgery (SRS)、複数回で行う場合にはstereotactic radiotherapy (SRT)という用語を用いるのが一般的である。

注2：現時点でSRTのエビデンスはないが、放射線生物学上SRTは有効性と安全性においてSRSに勝る。SRTを施行する場合の参考として、腫瘍径が＞3cmあるいは危険臓器が近接している場合には42Gy/7回を施行する[10]。

注3：RPA class Ⅲで予後が不良な場合、全脳照射20Gy/5回も考慮する。

8-2. 転移性骨腫瘍

1986年にイギリスにおいて30Gy/10回と8Gy/1回の比較試験において両者の除痛効果に差がないことが報告され、他のいくつかの無作為比較試験においても同様の結果が得られている[11〜13]。ASTRO evidence-based guidelineでは、ビホスホネート、Sr-89、手術的圧迫解除があっても放射線治療の必要性は変わらないこと、さまざまな分割方法があるが、長期コースの方が再照射を必要とする割合が低下することが示されている[14]。

また、即効性はないが、Sr-89、Rd-223は多発骨転移に有効な治療法である。Rd-223では疼痛の制御だけでなく、前立腺癌の多発骨転移に対して生存期間も延長させることは示されており、発売が待たれる[15]。

照射野の設定

局所

注：疼痛等で位置合わせの再現性は悪いのでPTVマージンは10mm以上が原則。しかし、肺や消化管などの障害を避けるためにマージンは臨機応変に決める。また、8Gy/1回法を行う場合は、原則的に3門以上の多門照射にて予期せぬ障害を起こさないよう十分な注意を払う。

推奨線量

8Gy/1回、20Gy/5回、30Gy/10回

8-3. 上大静脈症候群

緊急照射の適応とされるが、側副血行路のために重篤な症状を呈することはあまり経験しない。腫瘍が限局している時は、原発腫瘍に応じて肺癌やリンパ腫の項に準じて治療する[16]。すでに多発転移などが認められる姑息照射例では、30Gy/10回を投与する。

照射野の設定

上縦隔±原発巣±有意なリンパ節

推奨線量

姑息例：30Gy/10回
根治例：原発腫瘍の推奨線量を採用する

8-4. 脊髄圧迫

最も癌患者のQOLを低下させる病態の1つであるため、精力的に対応すべきである。Patchellの比較試験の結果からエントリー時に歩行可能な患者の歩行維持率（94% vs 74%）、歩行不能患者の歩行回復率（62% vs 19%）の両者において圧迫解除＋放射線治療が放射線治療単独より優れた成績が得られた[17]。施設の状況にもよるが、整形外科にコンサルトすることは必要である。Radesらは11の潜在的な危険因子を層別化したmatched pair studyを行った結果、運動機能、局所効果、生存において手術＋放射線治療と放射線治療単独はほとんど同等であると報告した[18]。また、Radesらは8Gy/1回、20Gy/5回、30Gy/10回、37.5Gy/15回、40Gy/20回で歩行機能の変化を比較した結果では有意差はなかったが、後ろの3者で照射野内再発率は低く、その後の比較試験で40Gy/20回と30Gy/10回では効果に有意差を認めなかった[19, 20]。

Radesらは脊髄圧迫改善の見通しを考える上で参考とな

るScoring System（点数が高いほど予後良好）を考案しているので参照して線量選択の参考にしてもよい[21]。

不全麻痺がある場合、糖尿病などの合併症が許せば、デカドロンを8〜16mg（分2）で投与し、4〜5日ごとに減量する。

照射野の設定

局所（転移性骨腫瘍に準じる）

推奨線量

30Gy／10回
予後不良例：8Gy／1回あるいは20Gy／5回
予後良好例：37.5Gy／15回

---

1) Gaspar L et al: Recursive partitioning analysis (RPA) of prognostic factors in three Radiation Therapy Oncology Group (RTOG) brain metastases trials. Int J Radiat Oncol Biol Phys 37(4): 745-751, 1997
2) Sperduto PW et al: Summary report on the graded prognostic assessment: an accurate and facile diagnosis-specific tool to estimate survival for patients with brain metastases. J Clin Oncol 30(4): 419-425, 2012
3) Patchell RA et al: Postoperative radiotherapy in the treatment of single metastases to the brain: a randomized trial. JAMA 280(17): 1485-1489, 1998
4) Andrews DW et al: Whole brain radiation therapy with or without stereotactic radiosurgery boost for patients with one to three brain metastases: phase Ⅲ results of the RTOG 9508 randomised trial. Lancet 363(9422): 1665-1672, 2004
5) Sperduto PW et al: Secondary analysis of RTOG 9508, a phase 3 randomized trial of whole-brain radiation therapy versus WBRT plus stereotactic radiosurgery in patients with 1-3 brain metastases; poststratified by the graded prognostic assessment (GPA). Int J Radiat Oncol Biol Phys 90(3): 526-531, 2014
6) Shaw E et al: Single dose radiosurgical treatment of recurrent previously irradiated primary brain tumors and brain metastases: final report of RTOG protocol 90-05. Int J Radiat Oncol Biol Phys 47(2): 291-298, 2000
7) Aoyama H et al: Stereotactic radiosurgery plus whole-brain radiation therapy vs stereotactic radiosurgery alone for treatment of

brain metastases: a randomized controlled trial. Jama 295(21): 2483-2491, 2006
8) Aoyama H et al: Stereotactic Radiosurgery With or Without Whole-Brain Radiotherapy for Brain Metastases: Secondary Analysis of the JROSG 99-1 Randomized Clinical Trial. JAMA Oncol 1(4): 457-464, 2015
9) Chang EL et al: Neurocognition in patients with brain metastases treated with radiosurgery or radiosurgery plus whole-brain irradiation: a randomised controlled trial. Lancet Oncol 10(11): 1037-1044, 2009
10) Tokuuye K et al: Fractionated stereotactic radiotherapy of small intracranial malignancies. Int J Radiat Oncol Biol Phys 42(5): 989-994, 1998
11) Hartsell WF et al: Randomized trial of short- versus long-course radiotherapy for palliation of painful bone metastases. J Natl Cancer Inst 97(11): 798-804, 2005
12) Foro Arnalot P et al: Randomized clinical trial with two palliative radiotherapy regimens in painful bone metastases: 30 Gy in 10 fractions compared with 8 Gy in single fraction. Radiother Oncol 89(2): 150-155, 2008
13) Kaasa S et al: Prospective randomised multicenter trial on single fraction radiotherapy (8 Gy x 1) versus multiple fractions (3 Gy x 10) in the treatment of painful bone metastases. Radiother Oncol 79(3): 278-284, 2006
14) Lutz S et al: Palliative radiotherapy for bone metastases: an ASTRO evidence-based guideline. Int J Radiat Oncol Biol Phys 79(4): 965-976, 2011
15) Parker C et al: Alpha emitter radium-223 and survival in metastatic prostate cancer. N Engl J Med 369(3): 213-223, 2013
16) Armstrong BA et al: Role of irradiation in the management of superior vena cava syndrome. Int J Radiat Oncol Biol Phys 13(4): 531-539, 1987
17) Patchell RA et al: Direct decompressive surgical resection in the treatment of spinal cord compression caused by metastatic cancer: a randomised trial. Lancet 366(9486): 643-648, 2005
18) Rades D et al: Matched pair analysis comparing surgery followed by radiotherapy and radiotherapy alone for metastatic spinal cord compression. J Clin Oncol 28(22): 3597-3604, 2010
19) Rades D et al: Evaluation of five radiation schedules and prognostic factors for metastatic spinal cord compression. J Clin Oncol 23(15): 3366-3375, 2005
20) Rades D et al: A prospective evaluation of two radiotherapy schedules with 10 versus 20 fractions for the treatment of metastatic spinal cord compression: final results of a multicenter

study. Cancer 101(11): 2687-2692, 2004
21) Rades D et al: Validation of a Score Predicting Post-Treatment Ambulatory Status After Radiotherapy for Metastatic Spinal Cord Compression. Int J Radiat Oncol Biol Phys 79(5): 1503-1506, 2011

memo

9. 皮膚癌

9-1. 皮膚悪性黒色腫

悪性度が高く、放射線感受性が低い腫瘍である。治療は広範切除術が主体で、切除断端を完全に陰性とすることが重要である。術後に小分割での放射線治療を行うことにより、局所制御率の向上が得られる可能性がある[1]。特に、リンパ節転移陽性例では術後に30Gy/5回/2.5週の放射線治療を行うことにより、局所制御の改善が得られ術後照射が推奨される[2]。イピリムマブ併用によりabscopal効果[3,4]が報告されており、局所療法としての放射線治療が全身療法としての役割をもつ可能性がある。

注：眼の脈絡膜悪性黒色腫は眼の項目を参照

照射野の設定

　局所±所属リンパ節領域

推奨線量

　術後照射：30Gy/5回、2回/週

9-2. 基底細胞癌・有棘細胞癌（扁平上皮癌）

一般に手術が優先されているが、手術拒否例で放射線治療は良い適応であり、治癒率は他の治療と同程度とされている[5]。切除例でも神経周囲浸潤陽性例およびリンパ節転移陽性例は術後照射の適応がある[6-8]。照射範囲は局所に1～2cmのマージンを設定する[9]。標準的な線量・分割法はないが50Gy/25Frから66Gy/33Frを周囲の要注意臓器や腫瘍の大きさによって決定する。術後照射は50Gy/25回を用いる。

照射野の設定

　局所＋1～2cm
　高リスク群ではリンパ節領域を含める

> 推奨線量

根治照射：66Gy/33回

術後照射：50Gy/25回

9-3. メルケル細胞癌

比較試験において手術単独よりも術後に放射線治療を施行することにより、局所制御率、無病生存率が向上することが示された[10]。データベースからの解析においても術後照射の有効性が報告されている[11, 12]。

照射線量は46Gyまではリンパ節領域を含め、完全切除例は50Gyまで、非完全切除例では56Gyまでが推奨される[13~15]。

> 照射野の設定

局所＋所属リンパ節領域

> 推奨線量

術後照射：50Gy/25回、非完全切除例は56Gy/28回

9-4. 血管肉腫

血管肉腫は頭皮に好発する。切除後に放射線治療を施行することにより局所制御率と生存率の向上が報告されている[16~18]。照射単独において70Gyの照射により局所制御率が得られる可能性が報告されている[19]。

曲面をもつ頭皮に対してVMATの有用性が報告されている[20]。当院においては^{192}Irを用いた小線源治療を施行している[21~23]。

> 照射野の設定

全頭皮

> 推奨線量

根治照射：70Gy/35回、小線源治療では60Gy/20回

9-5. 乳房外ページェット病

一般に手術が優先され、断端陽性例、深部浸潤例、リンパ節転移陽性例に対して放射線治療を施行される[24]が、照

射単独によっても良好な局所制御率が得られる可能性がある[25]。

> 照射野の設定

原発巣＋2～5cmおよび所属リンパ節領域

> 推奨線量

根治照射：60Gy/30回
術後照射：50Gy/25回

1) Stevens G et al: Locally advanced melanoma: results of postoperative hypofractionated radiation therapy. Cancer 88(1): 88-94, 2000
2) Agrawal S et al: The benefits of adjuvant radiation therapy after therapeutic lymphadenectomy for clinically advanced, high-risk, lymph node-metastatic melanoma. Cancer 115(24): 5836-5844, 2009
3) Stamell EF et al: The abscopal effect associated with a systemic anti-melanoma immune response. Int J Radiat Oncol Biol Phys 85(2): 293-295, 2013
4) Postow MA et al: Immunologic correlates of the abscopal effect in a patient with melanoma. N Engl J Med 366(10): 925-931, 2012
5) Neville JA et al: Management of nonmelanoma skin cancer in 2007. Nat Clin Pract Oncol 4(8): 462-469, 2007
6) Silverman MK et al: Recurrence rates of treated basal cell carcinomas. Part 4: X-ray therapy. J Dermatol Surg Oncol 18(7): 549-554, 1992
7) Voss N et al: Radiotherapy in the treatment of dermatologic malignancies. Dermatol Clin 16(2): 313-320, 1998
8) Warren TA et al: Outcomes after surgery and postoperative radiotherapy for perineural spread of head and neck cutaneous squamous cell carcinoma. Head Neck, 2014
9) Khan L et al: Recommendations for CTV margins in radiotherapy planning for non melanoma skin cancer. Radiother Oncol 104(2): 263-266, 2012
10) Jouary T et al: Adjuvant prophylactic regional radiotherapy versus observation in stage I Merkel cell carcinoma: a multicentric prospective randomized study. Ann Oncol 23(4): 1074-1080, 2012
11) Chen MM et al: The role of adjuvant therapy in the management of head and neck merkel cell carcinoma: an analysis of 4815 patients. JAMA Otolaryngol Head Neck Surg 141(2): 137-141, 2015
12) Mojica P et al: Adjuvant radiation therapy is associated with improved survival in Merkel cell carcinoma of the skin. J Clin Oncol

25(9): 1043-1047, 2007
13) Hruby G et al: The important role of radiation treatment in the management of Merkel cell carcinoma. Br J Dermatol 169(5): 975-982, 2013
14) Veness M et al: The role of radiotherapy alone in patients with merkel cell carcinoma: reporting the Australian experience of 43 patients. Int J Radiat Oncol Biol Phys 78(3): 703-709, 2010
15) Foote M et al: Effect of radiotherapy dose and volume on relapse in Merkel cell cancer of the skin. Int J Radiat Oncol Biol Phys 77(3): 677-684, 2010
16) Guadagnolo BA et al: Outcomes after definitive treatment for cutaneous angiosarcoma of the face and scalp. Head Neck 33(5): 661-667, 2011
17) Patel SH et al: Angiosarcoma of the scalp and face: the Mayo Clinic experience. JAMA Otolaryngol Head Neck Surg 141(4): 335-340, 2015
18) Pawlik TM et al: Cutaneous angiosarcoma of the scalp: a multidisciplinary approach. Cancer 98(8): 1716-1726, 2003
19) Ogawa K et al: Treatment and prognosis of angiosarcoma of the scalp and face: a retrospective analysis of 48 patients. Br J Radiol 85(1019): e1127-1133, 2012
20) Ostheimer C et al: The treatment of extensive scalp lesions using coplanar and non-coplanar photon IMRT: a single institution experience. Radiat Oncol 9: 82, 2014
21) Imai M et al: The 192Ir surface-mold technique for a whole scalp irradiation. J Jpn Soc Thre Radiol Oncol 11: 27-31, 1999
22) Nakamura R et al: Iridium-192 brachytherapy for hemorrhagic angiosarcoma of the scalp: a case report. Jpn J Clin Oncol 33(4): 198-201, 2003
23) Wittych J et al: Angiosarcoma of the scalp: a case report. J Contemp Brachytherapy 6(2): 208-212, 2014
24) Itonaga T et al: Radiotherapy in patients with extramammary Paget's disease--our own experience and review of the literature. Oncol Res Treat 37(1-2): 18-22, 2014
25) Hata M et al: Radiation therapy for extramammary Paget's disease: treatment outcomes and prognostic factors. Ann Oncol 25(1): 291-297, 2014

10. 骨軟部腫瘍

骨、筋肉、血管などの結合組織と呼ばれるものから発生した悪性腫瘍の総称である。骨軟部腫瘍には多様なものが含まれ、解剖学的にもさまざま、病理組織学的にもさまざまである。年齢もすべての年齢で起こりうるが、比較的若年者に多い。腫瘍の進行性もさまざまで急速に広がるものからゆっくりと進行するものまであるが、発見された時には10cm以上の巨大なものとなっていることもまれではない。放射線への感受性は低いものが多く、一般的には抵抗性である。

四肢に発生した場合は、四肢切断術が施行されることが多かったが、現在は腫瘍広範切除術と術前・術後の化学療法を併用し患肢温存を企図するようになってきた。放射線治療は、切除縁を縮小する保存的手術実施のための術前または術後照射として行われたり、あるいは切除縁不十分の場合の局所制御の向上を狙って術後照射として行われる。巨大腫瘍や切除困難な部位では根治的放射線治療が試みられるが、一般的な放射線治療の成績は不良であり、後述する粒子線治療の適応を考慮する[1-6]。病期分類による適応の違いは確立されていない。

10-1. 骨腫瘍

放射線治療の対象として比較的よく遭遇する腫瘍として、骨肉腫と脊索腫を概説する。

骨肉腫は代表的な骨の悪性腫瘍であり、放射線や化学療法は効きにくいとされる。近年、術前化学療法の進歩により、限局性の四肢原発骨肉腫の患肢温存率は80%に達しており、治癒切除例では10年生存率も60%以上が得られるようになってきた[3, 5]。しかし、骨盤や脊椎に発生すると機能障害を起こさずに外科切除することはきわめて困難である。そうした手術不能例では、放射線治療(＋化学療法)の5年生存率は10%以下であり、予後不良である。

脊索腫は、まれな腫瘍であり、頻度は骨軟部腫瘍の3%に

すぎないが粒子線治療で治せる難治性腫瘍として有名である。50%は仙骨から発生し、増大は緩徐であるが、発見時には12cm以上の巨大腫瘍を形成していることもまれではない[2]。仙骨脊索腫に対する一般的治療法は切除手術だが、第2仙椎より上位で完全切除すると直腸膀胱障害などを避けるのは困難であるため、機能障害を避ける上でも放射線治療が重要である。しかし、通常放射線治療では5年局所制御率が30%程度と低い。有効な化学療法はない。仙骨以外では頭蓋底からの発生が多い[6]。

骨腫瘍の組織型による放射線感受性は、Ewing肉腫＞巨細胞腫＞骨肉腫＞悪性線維性組織球腫（malignant fibrous histiocytoma: MFH）＞軟骨肉腫＞脊索腫とされるが、Ewing肉腫以外は、放射線抵抗性と考えて差し支えない。

CTVはGTVに3〜5cmのマージンをつけた範囲として設定し、50〜60Gy後のブースト照射では1〜3cmのマージンで設定する。

総線量はEwing肉腫で、55.8/31回〜60Gy/30回、その他の腫瘍で70Gy/35回を目標とするが、周囲の危険臓器（脊髄、消化管など）のため、十分な線量を投与できないことも多い。根治照射を行う際には、後述する粒子線の適応であるかどうかも検討すべきである[1〜3]。術後照射の線量は、高感受性腫瘍で50Gy/25回、低感受性腫瘍で66Gy/33回を目標とする。

照射野の設定
初期の照射野はGTV＋3〜5cm、ブースト照射はGTV＋1〜3cm

推奨線量
根治照射：Ewing肉腫55.8/31回〜60Gy/30回、その他70Gy/35回
術後照射：高感受性腫瘍50Gy/25回、低感受性腫瘍66Gy/33回

10-2. 軟部腫瘍

組織型による放射線感受性は、PNET (primitive neuroectodermal tumor) ＞ Ewing肉腫 ＞ 横紋筋肉腫 ＞ MFHの一部＞粘液型脂肪肉腫＞平滑筋肉腫＞円形細胞型脂肪肉腫＞＞紡錘形細胞型・多形性MFH＞線維肉腫といわれるが、PNET、Ewing肉腫、横紋筋肉腫(成人発生)以外は、放射線抵抗性と考えて差し支えない。照射法は、CTVはGTVに3～6cmのマージンをつけた範囲として設定し。筋膜でまとめられる関連筋群全体を含むように心がける。総線量はPNET、Ewing肉腫、横紋筋肉腫(成人発生)で、55.8/31回～60Gy/30回、その他の腫瘍で70Gy/35回/7週を目標とするが、周囲の危険臓器(脊髄、消化管など)のため、十分な線量を投与できないことも多い。根治照射を行う際には、後述する粒子線の適応であるかどうかも検討すべきである[4]。術後照射の線量は、高感受性腫瘍で50Gy/25回、低感受性腫瘍で66Gy/33回を目標とする。術後照射では術創を十分含める。

照射野の設定
初期の照射野はGTV＋3～6cm、ブースト照射を行う場合はGTV＋2～3cm

推奨線量
根治照射：高感受性腫瘍55.8/31回～60Gy/30回、低感受性腫瘍70Gy/35回
術後照射：高感受性腫瘍50Gy/25回、低感受性腫瘍66Gy/33回

10-3. 切除不能骨軟部腫瘍

骨・軟部腫瘍は、過去20年間、切除を基本とした集学的治療が最も成果を上げてきた疾患である。しかしながら、仙骨部肉腫を例にとると、切除が第一選択であるのは変わりないが、腫瘍の存在範囲によっては高位仙髄の切除が必要となり、排便排尿障害など術後の機能損失が大きい。手

術自体の侵襲も大きいため、特に高齢者に対しては負担の大きい治療である。また、発症した時点ですでに腫瘍が巨大なことも多く、切除適応とならない症例も多い。

放射線治療も最近では外部照射だけでなく小線源なども駆使され、四肢の骨軟部腫瘍で患肢温存等に重要な役割を果たしている[1]。しかし、本腫瘍は一般に放射線抵抗性であり、切除縁確保が困難で明らかな腫瘍残存を認める場合や、切除非適応となった症例での放射線の効果は不十分とされている。骨肉腫などの一部の組織型では化学療法が有効であるが、それだけでは局所療法として不十分である。粒子線治療は、その線量集中性により従来よりも高線量の投与が可能であり、放射線抵抗性の骨・軟部腫瘍に対しても有効であると期待される[2~6]。粒子線治療ではハーバード大、筑波大の頭蓋底脊索腫に対する陽子線治療成績[7,8]と放医研の体幹部骨軟部腫瘍に対する重粒子線治療の成績が有名である[1]。放医研では、第Ⅱ相試験から、粒子線治療により皮膚線量の低減を図る工夫をすることによりほとんど有害事象なく、5年局所制御率は79%、5生存率は61%と優れた成績が得られている[1]。頭蓋底発生を除く脊索腫95例においては、5年局所制御率が88%で、5年生存率は86%であった[2]。

1) Davis AM et al: Late radiotherapy mobidity following randomization to preoperative versus postoperative radiotherapy in extremity soft tissue sarcomas. Radiother Oncol 75(1): 48-53, 2005
2) Kamada T et al: Efficacy and safety of carbon ion radiotherapy in bone and soft tissue sarcomas. J Clin Oncol 20(22): 4466-4471, 2002
3) Imai R et al: Carbon ion radiotherapy for unresectable sacral chordomas. Clin Cancer Res 10(17): 5741-5746, 2004
4) Sugahara S et al: Carbon ion radiotherapy for localized primary sarcoma of the extremities: results of a phase I/Ⅱ trial. Radiother Oncol 105(2): 226-231, 2012
5) Serizawa I et al: Carbon ion radiotherapy for unresectable retroperitoneal sarcomas. Int J Radiat Oncol Biol Phys 75(1): 1105-1110, 2009

6) DeLaney TF et al: Radiotherapy for local control of osteosarcoma. Int J Radiat Oncol Biol Phys 61: 491-498, 2005
7) Munzenrider JE et al: Proton therapy for tumors of the skull base. Strahlenther Onkol 175 Suppl 2: 57-63, 1999
8) Igaki H et al: Clinical results of proton beam therapy for skull base chordoma. Int J Radiat Oncol Biol Phys 60(4): 1120-1126, 2004

memo

11. 小児

　小児腫瘍は、いずれもまれな腫瘍であり、晩期障害を避けるために細心の注意が必要である。たとえば、骨の成長障害を避けるために骨端線をはずす事や不妊を避けるために卵巣をブロック（外科と話し合ってあらかじめ照射野外になるように卵巣を移動させてもらうこともある）するなどの工夫が必要である。実際の治療では、症例ごとに国立成育医療センター（わが国で最も経験がある施設である）の放射線治療部にコンサルテーションして最新プロトコルに基づいて治療することが望ましい。

11-1. ウィルムス腫瘍

　わが国での症例数は年間約70～80例といわれているまれな腫瘍である。National Wilmus' Tumor Groupe (NWTSG)のランダム化比較試験の結果、治癒可能な腫瘍となっている[1~3]。現在はNWTSGの後を受けたCOG (Children's Oncology Group)プロトコルにそって治療を行うのが標準的である。強力な化学療法とともに予後良好群(Favorable Histology)のⅢ-Ⅳ期、びまん性退形成性腎芽腫の全病期、腎明細胞肉腫(Clear cell sarcoma of the kidney)の全病期、横紋筋腫瘍様肉腫(Rhabdoid tumor: RTK)の全病期が放射線治療の適応であり、術後照射を10.8Gy/6回/8日で行う。未分化腫瘍のⅢ期、RTKは予後不良なので19.8Gy/11回まで行う。術後照射は術後9日以内に開始するように定められている[1]。CTVは初診時に認められた腫瘍とリンパ節転移を含み、実際の照射野は1cm以上のマージンをつけるとともに側弯症を予防するために椎体全体を含む事が肝要である。腹膜播種が疑われる症例では、10.5Gy/7回の全腹腔照射（可能な限り大腿骨頭をブロック）を行う。

照射野の設定

術後照射：CTVは初診時に認められた腫瘍＋リンパ節転移巣（上記参照）

腹膜播種例：全腹腔照射

推奨線量

術後照射適応症例は、10.8Gy/6回（RTKなど19.8Gy/11回：上記参照）、全腹腔照射の場合10.5Gy/7回

11-2. 神経芽腫

小児固形癌の中では、最も頻度が高く、わが国では年間320例程度の発生数であるといわれている。年齢分布は0歳、次いで3歳にピークを示す二峰性のパターンを呈する1歳以下の症例は進行期にあっても長期生存の可能性が高く、自然退縮もあり得る。もう少し年長児（2歳以上）で発見されることが多い進行例は治療が困難なものが多い[4]。

わが国では、病期分類に日本小児外科学会悪性腫瘍委員会分類が用いられる。予後不良因子として腫瘍細胞の染色体数が2倍体、MYCN遺伝子の増幅、trk A遺伝子の低発現、血清NSE（Neuron specific enolase）の高値、が挙げられる[4]。予後不良因子をもつ進行神経芽腫の治療法は、初診時に開腹生検を施行して組織診断とともに病理組織の嶋田分類[5]、遺伝子検索が行われる。この後、シスプラチンを中心とした導入化学療法が3～4コース行われ、縮小したところで原発巣の切除とリンパ節郭清が行われ、この後、術後照射が行われる[6]。骨転移を伴う高リスク症例などでは、造血幹細胞移植を前提とした骨髄破壊的な化学療法も行われる[7]。こうして高リスクの進行神経芽腫でも治癒する症例がでてきている。骨転移部には化学療法と併行して19.8Gy/11回の放射線治療が行われる。

照射野は、小児外科医の術中の腫瘍進展範囲の情報に基づいて手術前の原発巣とリンパ節転移に臨床的なマージン（1.0～1.5cm）をとってCTVを形成する。年齢により線量は

異なり、1歳以下は19.8Gy/11回、2歳までは25.2Gy/14回、2歳以上30.6Gy/17回である。骨髄破壊的な化学療法を行う場合は線量を減量でき19.8Gy/11回（肉眼的残存病巣へはさらに10.8Gy/6回ブースト照射）でよい。線量制約は、肝臓の50％以上が9Gy未満、健側腎臓の50％以上が8Gy未満となるようにする。

照射野の設定

術後照射：手術前の原発巣とリンパ節転移、ブースト照射を行う場合は肉眼的残存病巣

推奨線量

術後照射適応症例は1歳以下：19.8Gy/11回
2歳まで：25.2Gy/14回
2歳以上：30.6Gy/17回
骨髄破壊的な化学療法を行う場合：19.8Gy/11回（肉眼的残存病巣へはさらに10.8Gy/6回ブースト照射）
骨転移巣：19.8Gy/11回

11-3. 横紋筋肉腫

わが国での症例数は年間約90症例といわれている。横紋筋肉腫は筋膜にそって進展し、浸潤性が強い。手術だけでは局所再発を来しやすく放射線治療と化学療法を加えた集学的治療が必要である。Intergroup Rhabdomyosarcoma Study (IRS) による臨床研究が有名であり[8〜11]、IRS-Vのプロトコルにそって治療されることが多いが[10, 11]、日本横紋筋肉腫研究グループ (JRSG) のガイドラインも取り入れられつつある。組織型は胎児型 (Embryonal type) と胞巣型 (Alveolar type) に分けられ、胞巣型は予後不良である。

IRSによる臨床分類では、Group Ⅰ（組織学的完全切除）、Group Ⅱ（顕微鏡的術後残存）、Group Ⅲ（肉眼的腫瘍残存）、Group Ⅳ（遠隔転移、悪性胸膜水、播種のいずれかを伴う）に分けられ、Group Ⅰの胞巣型およびGroup Ⅱは、41.4Gy/23回の術後照射を必要とする。Group Ⅲでは、眼窩で

45Gy/25回、その他の部位で50.4Gy/28回を照射する。照射開始時期は術後化学療法開始後3週目である。GTVは原発病巣＋腫大リンパ節で、CTVはGTV＋1.5cmで開始する。照射法は骨格系の変形を避けるために、椎体全体を照射野に入れるなどの均等な線量投与を心がける。その結果、前後対向2門などの単純な照射法が選択されることが多い。照射野が大きくなる場合は1回線量を1.5Gyにしたり、36～41.4Gyで照射野を縮小するなどの工夫が必要である。小児での正常組織の耐容線量は、IRS-Vプロトコルに掲載されているので、この耐容線量を超えないように治療計画を立てる。小児において41.4Gyは晩期障害を避け得るぎりぎりの線量であり、常に合併症を念頭に置く必要ある。

照射野の設定

原発病巣＋腫大リンパ節＋1.5cmが原則（上記参照）

推奨線量

術後照射：Group Ⅰの胞巣型およびGroup Ⅱは41.4Gy/23回。Group Ⅲは眼窩で45Gy/25回、その他の部位で50.4Gy/28回。

1) Green DM: The treatment of stages I-Ⅳ favorable histology Wilms' tumor. J Clin Oncol 22(6): 1366-1372, 2004
2) Green DM et al: Comparison between single-dose and divided-dose administration of dactinomycin and doxorubicin for patients with Wilms' tumor: a report from the National Wilms' Tumor Study Group. J Clin Oncol 16(1): 237-245, 1998
3) Dome JS et al: The treatment of anaplastic histology Wilms' tumor: a results from the fifth National Wilms' Tumor Study Group. J Clin Oncol 24(15): 2352-2358, 2006
4) Maris JM: Recnt advances in Neuroblastom. N Engl J Med 362(23): 2202-2011, 2010
5) Shimada H et al: The International Neuroblastoma Pathology Classification for prognostic evaluation of patiients with peripheral neuroblastic tumors: a report from the Children's Cancer Group. Cancer 92(9): 2451-2461, 2001
6) Castleberry RP et al: Radiotherapy improves the outlook for patients older than 1 year with Pediatric Oncology Group stage C

neuroblastoma. J Clin Oncol 9(5): 789-795, 1991
7) Bradfield SM et al: Fractionated low-dose radiotherapy after myeloablative stem cell transplantation for local control in patients with high-risk neuroblastoma. Cancer 100(6): 1268-1275, 2004
8) Wolden SL et al: Indications for radiotherapy and chemotherapy after complete resection in rhabdomyosarcoma: A report from the Intergroup Rhabdomyosarcoma Studies I to Ⅲ. J Clin Oncol 17(11): 3468-3475, 1999
9) Crist WM et al: Intergroup rhabdomyosarcoma study-IV: results for patients with nonmetastatic disease. J Clin Oncol 19(12): 3091-3102, 2001
10) Raney RB et al: The Intergroup Rhabdomyosarcoma Study Group (IRSG) : Major Lessons From the IRS-I Through IRS-IV Studies as Background for the current IRS-V Treatment Protocols. Sarcoma 5(1): 9-15, 2001
11) Raney RB et al: Results of the Intergroup Rhabdomyosarcoma Study Group D9602 protocol, using vincristine and dactinomycin with or without cyclophosphamideand radiation therapy, for newly diagnosed patients with low-risk embryonal rhabdomyosarcoma: a report from the Soft Tissue Sarcoma Comimittee of the Children's Oncology group. J Clin Oncol 29(10): 1312-1318, 2011

12. 良性疾患

12-1. 脳動静脈奇形
(AVM：Arteriovenous malformation)

　脳AVMは随伴する動脈瘤が破綻して年間2～4%の頻度で出血を来すことが知られており、この出血予防が目的である[1]。脳AVMの治療は手術の摘出が第1選択であるが、手術リスクが高い症例では放射線治療が選択される。保存的な治療としては血管塞栓術があり、単独治療のほか、術前や照射前にも行われる[1]。

　CTV=GTV=nidusである。先行して行われた血管造影の所見を参考にして造影CT上でnidusを設定し、PTVは1mmマージンとする。1回照射で行われる定位手術的照射(SRS)では、辺縁線量20Gyが用いられることが多い。閉塞するのには1～5年程度が必要であり、閉塞率は70～80%である[2]。定位放射線治療を行うことで、出血既往者の治療後潜伏期における出血のリスクは減少すると示されている[3]。出血の既往のない患者に対するARUBA trialの結果は、医学的管理のみの経過観察の方が死亡、出血のリスクが少ないことが示された[4]。慎重に治療の適応を決定する必要がある。

　nidusの長径>28mm、体積≧4.5cm^2、V_{12}≧20cm^{2}で放射線治療後合併症のリスクとなるとの報告もあり[5]、nidusが3cmを超える大きさの場合は、照射前塞栓術によってCTVを小さくできないかどうかの検討も必要である。血管閉塞という放射線による反応に期待した治療法であるので、分割照射にする理論的な意味はないが、nidusが大きな症例では分割照射の方が安全と考えられる。

　北大では、75個のうち33個のeloquent regionに位置するか、2.5cm以上の場合4回に分割照射するSRTを施行し、それ以外の42個のAVMに対してはSRSを施行した。患者背景が異なるためにSRSとSRTの比較はできないが、彼らは安全な治療のためにこのような層別化を提案している[6]。

照射野の設定

局所(Nidus)

推奨線量

SRS：20Gy/1回
SRT：34Gy/4回

12-2. ケロイド

ピアス、外傷、痤瘡、水痘等が発生要因となり、好発部位は胸骨部、肩甲骨部、恥骨上部、耳垂である。美容的問題のほか、疼痛、掻痒のため、精神的な苦痛を受けている患者も多い。術後照射として行われ[7, 8]、術前に形成外科医と照射が可能な部位かどうかを打ち合わせておく。術創の周囲に5〜10mmのマージンをつけ照射野を設定し、4〜6MeV電子線を用いて5〜10mmのボーラスをおいて80%線量が皮膚表面より1cm以下になるように深さを調整する。照射は術翌日から術後72時間以内に開始する[9]。線量は12〜20Gyが用いられるが、本書では12Gy/3回/3日を投与する[8]。張力のかかりやすい部位に再発しやすく胸骨部、肩、恥骨上部では、16Gy/4回/4日に増やしてもよい。2次発癌が問題と考えられるが、通常使われる10〜20Gyでの2次発癌発生の報告はない[10]。

照射野の設定

術創に5〜10mmのマージンをつけて設定し、4〜6MeV電子線で5〜10mmのボーラスをおく。

推奨線量

12Gy/3回

12-3. 甲状腺眼症

副腎皮質ホルモン治療が第一選択で、無効例に対してや副腎皮質ホルモン治療との併用療法として行う[11]。CTVは外眼筋と眼球後軟部組織で実質的に眼窩照射となる[12, 13]。

照射野の設定

CTVは外眼筋と眼球後部組織、側方から5度程度ビームを傾けるなどして、直接の水晶体への照射を極力避ける。

推奨線量

20Gy/10回

---

1) Ogilvy CS et al: AHA Scientific Statement: Recommendations for the management of intracranial arteriovenous malformations: a statement for healthcare professionals from a special writing group of the Stroke Council, American Stroke Association. Stroke 32(6): 1458-1471, 2001
2) Flickinger JC et al: A multi-institutional analysis of complication outcomes after arteriovenous malformation radiosurgery. Int J Radiat Oncol Biol Phys 44(1): 67-74, 1999
3) Maruyama K et al: The risk of hemorrhage after radiosurgery for cerebral arteriovenous malformations. N Engl J Med 352(2): 146-1534, 2005
4) Mohr JP et al: Medical management with or without interventional therapy for unruptured brain arteriovenous malformations(ARUBA): a multicentre, non-blinded, randomised trial. Lancet 383(9917): 614-621, 2014
5) Herbert C et al: Factors Predictive of Symptomatic Radiation Injury AfterLinear Accelerator-Based Stereotactic Radiosurgery forIntracerebral Arteriovenous Malformations.Int J Radiat Oncol Biol Phys 83(3): 872-877, 2012
6) Chang TC et al: Stereotactic irradiation for intracranial arteriovenous malformation using stereotactic radiosurgery or hypofractionated stereotactic radiotherapy. Int J Radiat Oncol Biol Phys 60(3): 861-870, 2004
7) Botwood N et al: The risks of treating keloids with radiotherapy. Br J Radiol 72(864): 1222-1224, 1999
8) Sclafani AP et al: Prevention of earlobe keloid recurrence with postoperative corticosteroid injections versus radiation therapy: a randomized, prospective study and review of the literature. Dermatol Surg 22(6): 569-574, 1996
9) Lee SY et al: Postoperative electron beam radiotherapy for keloids: treatment outcome and factors associated with occurrence and recurrence. Ann Dermatol 27(1): 53-58, 2015
10) Leer JW et al: Indications and treatment schedules for irradiation of benign diseases: a survey. Radiother Oncol 48(3): 249-257, 1998
11) Abboud M et al: Outcome of thyroid associated ophthalmopathy treated by radiation therapy. Radiat Oncol 6: 46, 2011

12) Petersen IA et al: Prognostic factors in the radiotherapy of Graves' ophthalmopathy. Int J Radiat Oncol Biol Phys 19(2): 259-264, 1990
13) Mourits MP et al: Radiotherapy for Graves' orbitopathy: randomised placebo-controlled study. Lancet 355(9214): 1505-1509, 2000

memo

参考資料

・耐容線量

1991年にEmamiらが部分耐容線量の概念を提唱し、それを照射体積との関連で示したデータは現在においても有用であり、現在でも用いられている。しかし、臨床データは積み重ねられており、これだけで耐容線量を考えている人はもはやいない。2010年にMarksらは3次元治療計画時代に有効に使用できる臓器ごとの線量・体積・有害事象の確率の関係を示したデータ（Quantitative analysis of normal tissue effects in the clinic：QUANTEC）を提示した。このデータも完成されたものではなく、正しく適応されなければならないことはいうまでもない。ここでは、現在においても用いられているEmamiの表とQUANTECの表に加えて、耐容線量が低く、成長障害を考慮する必要がある小児の耐容線量についてはIRS-Vに準拠した小児の耐容線量を示した。

Emamiの耐容線量表

体積	TD 5/5 (Gy)			判定基準
	1/3	2/3	3/3	
大腿骨頭			52	壊死
顎関節	65	60		開口障害
肋骨	50			病的骨折
脳	60	50	45	壊死
脳幹	60	53	50	壊死
視神経		50		失明
視交叉		50		失明
脊髄	50 (5cm)	50 (10cm)	47 (20cm)	脊髄症
馬尾		60		神経損傷
腕神経叢	62	61	60	神経損傷
水晶体		10		白内障
網膜		45		失明
中耳・外耳		30		急性漿液性耳炎
		55		慢性漿液性耳炎
耳下腺		32		口内乾燥症
喉頭	79	70		軟骨壊死
		45		喉頭浮腫

臓器	TD 5/5 (Gy)			判定基準
肺	45	30	17.5	肺臓炎
心臓	60	45	40	心外膜炎
食道	60	58	55	狭窄、穿孔
胃	60	55	50	潰瘍、穿孔
小腸	50		40	閉塞、穿孔
大腸	55		45	閉塞、穿孔、潰瘍
直腸			60	直腸炎、壊死、狭窄
肝臓	50	35	30	肝不全
腎臓	50	30	23	腎炎
膀胱		80	65	膀胱萎縮

(Emami B et al: Tolerance of normal tissue to therapeutic irradiation. Int J Radiat Oncol Biol Phys 21(1): 109-122, 1991 より改変)

Quantitative analysis of normal tissue effect in the clinic (QUANTEC)

臓器		線量体積関係	発生率(%)	エンドポイント	備考
脳	3DCRT	Dmax＜60	＜3	症候性脳壊死	
		Dmax＝72	5		
		Dmax＝90	10		
	SRS	V12＜5-10cc	＜20		
脳幹		全体に＜54Gy	＜5	恒久的脳神経症	
		D1-10cc≦59			
	SRS	Dmax＜12.5Gy			
視神経、交叉	3DCRT	Dmax＜55Gy	＜3	視神経症	
		Dmax 55Gy-60Gy	3-7		
		Dmax＞60Gy	＞7-20		
	SRS	Dmax＜12Gy	＜10		
脊髄	3DCRT	Dmax＝50	0.2	脊髄症	
		Dmax＝60	6		
		Dmax＝69	50		
	SRS	Dmax＝13	1		
	SRT (hypofraction)	Dmax＝20	1		
内耳	3DCRT	Mean dose≦45	＜30	聴力喪失	
	SRS	処方線量≦14	＜25		
耳下腺	3DCRT	両側Mean dose＜25	＜20	唾液分泌低下 (＜25%)	
		片側Mean dose＜20	＜20		
		両側Mean dose＜39	＜50		

臓器		線量体積関係	発生率(%)	エンドポイント	備考
咽頭(咽頭筋)	3DCRT	Mean dose＜50	＜20	嚥下困難、誤嚥	
喉頭	3DCRT	Dmax＝66	＜20	発声機能喪失	化療併用
		Mean dose＜50	＜30	誤嚥	
		Mean dose＜44	＜20	浮腫	
		V50＜27%			
肺	3DCRT	V20≦30%	＜20	症候性放射線肺臓炎	
		Mean dose＝7	5		
		Mean dose＝13	10		
		Mean dose＝20	20		
		Mean dose＝24	30		
		Mean dose＝27	40		
食道	3DCRT	Mean dose＜34	5-20	急性食道炎(G3)	
		V35＜50%	＜30	急性食道炎(G2)	
		V50＜40%			
		V70＜20%			
心臓	3DCRT	Mean dose＜26Gy	＜15	心外膜炎	
		V30＜46%			
		V25＜10%	＜1	長期心臓死	
肝	3DCRT	Mean dose＜30-32Gy	＜5	肝不全	正常肝
		Mean dose＜42	＜50		
		Mean dose＜28	＜5		Child A
		Mean dose＜36	＜50		
	SBRT 3 fractions	Mean dose＜13Gy	＜5		原発肝癌
	SBRT 6 fractions	Mean dose＜18Gy			
	SBRT 3 fractions	Mean dose＜15Gy			肝転移
	SBRT 6 fractions	Mean dose＜20Gy			
	正常肝＞700cc	Dmax＜15Gy			3-5 fractions
腎	3DCRT	Mean dose＜15-18Gy	＜5	臨床的腎不全	
		Mean dose＜28Gy	＜50		
		V12＜55%	＜5		
		V20＜32%			
		V23＜30%			
		V28＜20%			
胃	3DCRT	D100＜44	＜7	潰瘍	

臓器		線量体積関係	発生率(%)	エンドポイント	備考
小腸	3DCRT	V15<120cc	<10	G3以上	化療併用
		V45<195cc			
直腸	3DCRT	V50<50%	<15	G2以上晩期毒性	
			<10	G3以上晩期毒性	
		V60<35%	<15	G2以上晩期毒性	
			<10	G3以上晩期毒性	
		V65<25%	<15	G2以上晩期毒性	
			<10	G3以上晩期毒性	
		V70<20%	<15	G2以上晩期毒性	
			<10	G3以上晩期毒性	
		V75<15%	<15	G2以上晩期毒性	
			<10	G3以上晩期毒性	
膀胱	3DCRT	Dmax<65	<6	G3 late RTOG	
		V65≦50%			
		V70≦35%			
		V75≦25%			
		V80≦15%			
尿道球	3DCRT	Mean dose<50Gy	<35	勃起機能不全	
		D90<50	<35		
		D60-70<70	<55		

(Marks LB et al: Use of normal tissue complication probability models in the clinic. Int J Radiat Oncol Biol Phys 76(3 Suppl): S10-19, 2010 より改変)

IRS-Vに準拠した小児の耐容線量

危険臓器	耐容線量
両腎	14.4Gy
全肝	23.4Gy
両肺	14.4Gy
全脳 3歳超	30.6Gy
全脳 3歳以下	23.4Gy
視神経および視交叉	46.8Gy
脊髄	45.0Gy
消化管	45.0Gy
全腹腔	30.0Gy/20回
全心臓	30.6Gy
水晶体	14.4Gy
涙腺	41.4Gy

頭頸部のリンパ節領域

　リンパ節領域を下表のごとく定義して、原発巣、リンパ節転移の状況から顕微鏡的な転移の範囲をデータに基づいて推測する。強度変調放射線治療の登場により、照射が必要と考えられる領域に必要と思われる線量を投与するとともに、重要臓器の線量を耐容線量以下に抑えるという治療が可能となった。(Som PM et al: Imaging-based nodal classification for evaluation of neck metastatic adenopathy. AJR Am J Roentgenol 174(3): 837-844, 2000 の図を参考にすると理解しやすい)

レベル	頭側	尾側	前方	後方	外側	内側
Ia	下顎骨下縁	舌骨	広頸筋	舌骨	顎二腹筋	(—)
Ib	顎下腺	舌骨	広頸筋	顎下腺後縁	下顎骨	顎二腹筋
IIa	C1横突起	舌骨下縁	顎下腺後縁	内頸静脈後縁	SCMN	内頸動脈内側
IIb	C1横突起	舌骨下縁	内頸静脈後縁	SCMN後縁	SCMN	深頸筋群
III	舌骨下縁	輪状軟骨下縁	SCMN前縁	SCMN後縁	SCMN	深頸筋群
IV	輪状軟骨	鎖骨	SCMN前縁	SCMN後縁	SCMN	傍脊椎筋群
Va	舌骨上縁	輪状軟骨下縁	SCMN後縁	僧帽筋	広頸筋	傍脊椎筋群
Vb	輪状軟骨下縁	鎖骨	SCMN後縁	僧帽筋	広頸筋	傍脊椎筋群
VI	甲状腺	胸骨柄	皮膚	食道/気管間	SCMN内縁	気管

SCMN：胸鎖乳突筋

(Levendag P et al: Intraoperative validation of CT-based lymph nodal levels, sublevels IIa and IIb: is it of clinical use in selective radiation therapy? Int J Radiat Oncol Biol Phys 62(3): 690-699, 2005 を改変)

強度変調放射線治療を始めるにあたって

　通常の3次元治療は最適と思われる照射門、各門ごとの投与線量を決定し、線量分布を計算する。その線量分布が妥当であると判断すれば治療を開始し、妥当でないと判断されれば妥当と判断されるまで試行錯誤を繰り返すという

ものである。これに対して、強度変調放射線治療は腫瘍に照射すべき線量、重要臓器に線量・体積関係（限界となる線量とその線量が許される体積）を処方し、コンピュータにより設定した照射方法を実現するための照射方法を逆計算して各照射門の投与線量を決定する方法である。考え方の逆転であり、コペルニクス的転回といえる。ここで出てきた解は、各照射門の不均質な線量分布であるが、全門の線量分布を足し合わせるとより理想に近づいた線量分布となる。ここで求められるのは、最適な腫瘍照射線量と重要臓器の照射線量の限界についての臨床データである。また、化学療法が加わる場合には、その修飾によりさらに複雑となる。下記に頭頸部癌のリンパ節の照射範囲を決定するための参考資料を示す。

原発巣、臨床的にリンパ節転移の有無による転移病巣の頻度

	ルビエール		Level I		Level II		Level III		Level IV		Level V	
	N-	N+	N-	N+	N-	N+	N-	N+	N-	N+	N-	N+
上咽頭	40	86										
口腔												
舌			14	39	19	73	16	27	3	11	0	0
口腔底			16	72	12	51	7	29	2	11	0	5
			25	38	19	84	6	25	5	10	1	4
中咽頭												
舌根	0	6	4	19	30	89	22	22	7	10	0	18
扁桃	4	12	0	8	19	74	14	31	9	16	0	12
下咽頭												
咽頭壁	16	21	0	11	9	84	18	72	0	40	0	20
梨状窩	0	9	0	2	15	77	8	57	0	23	0	22
喉頭												
上部	0	4	6	2	18	70	18	48	9	17	2	16
声門			0	9	21	42	29	71	7	24	7	2

Chao KS et al: Determination and delineation of nodal target volumes for head-and-neck cancer based on patterns of failure in patients receiving definitive and postoperative IMRT. Int J Radiat Oncol Biol Phys 53(5): 1174-1184, 2002 より

医学生が知っておくべき放射線治療の知識

医学生を対象として、医師国家試験出題基準の用語解説と各論において放射線治療関連で出題されそうな箇所を取

り上げた。さらに学ぶには、上述したマニュアルを読むとともに、取り上げた参考文献を読まれることをお勧めする。

医師国家試験出題基準に取り上げられているキーワードの解説

●医学総論

A. 放射線感受性

放射線感受性と放射線反応性とは異なる。たとえば、中枢神経悪性リンパ腫は生存中央値が2年に届かないきわめて悪性の腫瘍である。しかし、初期効果はよく、放射線治療により腫瘍は一旦縮小、消失し症状も改善するが、すぐに再発する。これは、放射線の反応性はよいが、感受性が悪い例である。

A-1 正常組織の放射線感受性

一般に分裂頻度が高いものは感受性が高く、低いものは低い。これがベルゴニートリボンドーの法則である。また、形態的、機能的に未分化な細胞は感受性が高い。例外も多いが、放射線感受性を推測する上で役立つ法則である。

A-2 腫瘍の放射線感受性

腫瘍の組織型、分化度が大きく影響する。高感受性組織から発生した腫瘍は高感受性の傾向をもつ。

A-3 放射線治療可能比

正常組織耐容線量／腫瘍致死線量と定義され、これが高いほど治療がしやすい。

B. 放射線効果の修飾

B-1 酸素効果

低酸素状態では放射線感受性が低くなる。これを数値化したものが酸素効果比(oxygen enhancement ratio：OER)で、低酸素下での等効果線量／酸素下での等効果線量で表す。

B-2 放射線増感剤

放射線と同時に投与された時にその効果を高める薬剤。代表的なものに低酸素状態が存在する腫瘍組織に対して酸

素類似の効果を示すミソニダゾール(Misonidazol)があるが、臨床試験で有効性は証明されていない。

B-3 温熱効果

熱に対する細胞の生存曲線は放射線のそれと類似している。しかし、低酸素状態にある細胞は栄養欠乏状態にあるために熱に対する感受性が高くなる。このため、放射線治療との併用は有効である。

B-4 細胞周期

放射線感受性は細胞周期によって変化する。G2、M期で感受性が高く、S期の終わりとG1初期が低い。

B-5 線エネルギー付与 (LET)

放射線が飛程の単位長さあたりに周囲に付与するエネルギー。これが高いほど生物学的効果比(relative biological effectiveness RBE)が高くなり、低酸素状態においても殺細胞効果が高まるためOERが低くなる。

B-6 線量率

単位時間当たりに与える線量。

C. 空間的線量分布

表示法として深部線量百分率、等線量曲線がある。

C-1 深部線量百分率

組織の吸収線量を深さの関数としてプロットしたもの。

C-2 等線量曲線

等高線のように等線量領域を結んだ図。

C-3 線量計算

吸収線量を計算により求めること。さまざまな計算アルゴリズムが開発、改善されて、精度が向上している。

C-4 標的体積の決定

照射の標的となる体積。臨床標的体積とは腫瘍のミクロの進展も考慮に入れて、照射すべき体積であり、これを実現するためにこれにマージンをつけて照射する。

D. 時間的線量配分

一般に1回で照射する1回照射よりも何回にも分けて照射する分割照射の方が放射線生物学的に効果的とされ、これが標準となっている。最適な分割方法は、腫瘍の生物的特徴などのさまざまな因子により異なる。

D-1 回復・再増殖・再酸素化・再分布（4R）

放射線生物学でいう4Rに回復（repair）、再増殖（repopulation）、再酸素化（reoxygenation）、再分布（redistribution）がある。放射線治療はこれらの現象を巧みに利用して、治療効果を上げるものである。大量の放射線が当たると細胞は致死障害を受けるが、その手前の量では回復可能な亜致死障害にとどまる。このときの腫瘍より正常組織の回復が早いことを利用して治療するのが分割照射である。放射線治療において治療期間が長くなると効きが悪くなるのは治療中においても腫瘍が再増殖するためである。腫瘍の中心部は低酸素状態になっており、放射線治療の効果が低下する。放射線をあてて腫瘍の外側の効きがよい酸素化領域の細胞が死滅脱落すると、低酸素領域であった場所にも酸素がいきわたるようになる。この部分が酸素化領域になって、放射線が効きやすくなる。分割照射は次々と酸素化領域に代えていくことにより効果的な治療となる。細胞周期により放射線の感受性が変化する。最初の照射で感受性の高い周期の細胞が死滅するために細胞の周期が一定の状態になる。これを再分布と呼ぶ。時間をおいてこれらの細胞が感受性の高い周期に移動したとき照射すれば効率よく治療することができる。

D-2 通常分割照射

1回2Gy程度の線量を毎日照射する方法。

D-3 多分割照射

放射線生物学でいう回復の現象を利用して、治療期間を変えずに分割回数を増やし、総線量を増やすことによって正常組織の有害反応を増加することなく抗腫瘍効果を上げることを期待する方法。例）1回線量を1.2Gy、1日2回、総

線量72Gyでは、通常の1日1回2Gy、総線量60Gyの通常治療と同じ6週間で72Gyに線量を上げることができる。

D-4 少(寡)分割照射

1回線量を高くして治療期間を減らすことによって、腫瘍の再増殖を抑えて治療効果を高めようとする方法。

E. 装置と治療技術

E-1 外照射

体の外からX線電子線、粒子線などの放射線を照射する治療方法で、一般にリニアックが用いられている。

E-1-1 画像誘導放射線治療(IGRT)

画像技術を用いて正確な位置合わせをして高精度の照射を実現する方法。

E-1-2 定位放射線治療

小腫瘍に対して正確な画像計測を行って、3次元的に一点に放射線を集中して腫瘍に高線量を投与し、周囲の正常組織の線量を減らす方法。

E-1-3 強度変調放射線治療(IMRT)

照射方法を決めてからその方法で得られる線量分布の是非を評価するという従来のが従来の方法であった。これに対してIMRTは、腫瘍への投与線量を処方するとともに周囲の正常組織の線量制約を定め、コンピュータでこれを実現するための最適解を逆計算して設定する方法であり、原理的に考えると究極的な治療計画法である。これにより、さらに優れた線量分布が得られるようになった。

E-1-4 重粒子線治療

重粒子とは陽子あるいはそれ以上の重い粒子。この代表である陽子線、炭素線にはブラッグピークという、エネルギーに対応した一定の深さで吸収線量のピークが生じるという特性がある。これと腫瘍を一致させれば、腫瘍に高線量、周囲の組織に低線量の照射が可能となる。

E-2 密封小線源治療

放射線同位元素を密封した線源を用いて、腫瘍に高線量

を投与する治療法。距離の二乗に反比例して線量が低減するため、線源の近くに存在する腫瘍には高線量が照射され、遠くに位置する正常組織の線量が低減するという優れた線量集中性をもつ。

E-3 放射線同位元素 (RI) 内用療法 (内照射療法、内部照射療法)

放射線同位元素を目的の組織に集積させ、その内部から治療しようとする方法。代用的なものに甲状腺癌のI-131療法、Sr-89療法がある。前者は、I-131は甲状腺細胞に特異的に取り込まれ、そこから出され飛程の短いベータ線により治療するものであり、甲状腺に集中的に治療することができる。特に、甲状腺癌の多発肺転移では有効性が高い。良性疾患のバセドウ病に対しても内用療法の適応がある。後者は、Caの代わりに骨に取り込まれ、同じく飛程の短いベータ線で治療するもので、多発骨転移に対する有効な治療法である。

E-4 治療の質と安全管理

F. 放射線治療の適応

放射線治療の特長は適応範囲が広いことにある。部位別には頭頂から足先まで適応となり、小児から高齢者において手術が不可能な状態においても適応で、根治治療から姑息治療まで幅が広い。この理由は放射線が局所療法であり全身的な影響が少ないことによる。

F-1 根治的照射

治癒を目的とした照射。腫瘍全体を照射範囲に含み、腫瘍を制御できる線量を投与できることが必要である。

F-2 準根治的照射

臨床的に見て治癒を期待できないが、照射体積の腫瘍が根絶されると仮定すれば治癒する可能性のある照射。

F-3 対症的照射

延命あるいは、疼痛や出血などの症状を緩和する目的で行う照射。

G. 集学的治療

手術療法、化学療法、ホルモン療法などのいくつかの治療を組み合わせて効果を上げようとする治療法である。

G-1 術前・術中・術後（周術期）照射

術前照射は手術前に照射することにより、腫瘍の切除を容易にし、腫瘍切除の根治度を上げて治療成績の向上を図ろうとする治療法。術後照射は、術後に残存していることが予想される範囲に照射することによって再発率を下げて治療成績の向上に結びつけようとする治療法で、手術所見を加味して照射範囲を決定できるので無駄な照射を減らせるという利点をもつ。術中照射は、術中に照射したくない消化管などを避けて照射できるという利点をもつと同時に、1回で照射せざるを得ないという欠点をもつ。

G-2 化学療法との併用

化学放射線療法は多くの局所進行癌（腫瘍学的に手術の適応がないが、局所に腫瘍が留まっている状態）に対して、有効性が示されている。今後は分子標的薬剤との併用が期待される。

H. 照射の有害反応

放射線治療の効果がでるには時間がかかるのと同様に有害反応が出るのにも時間がかかる。この中で放射線治療中にでる初期有害反応の機序は炎症であるので、治療後は治癒する。これに対して治療が終わってしばらくしてから出現する遅発性有害反応の機序は変性であるためにしばしば進行性である。したがって、放射線治療はこの遅発性有害反応を起こさないように治療をする必要がある。

●医学各論

放射線治療がそれぞれの領域でどのような位置を占めているかという「癌治療の中の放射線治療」という考え方が必要である。

1)脳腫瘍

放射線抵抗性の多形成膠芽腫の治療は腫瘍を可能な限り摘出する。これにより、症状の改善が得られ、病理が確定する。術後照射として残存腫瘍に対してテモゾロマイド同時併用による化学放射線治療を施行する。MGMTプロモータにメチル化が生じている場合が良好な予後因子であり、長期生存例にIDHの変異例が多いと報告されている。

胚芽腫は化学療法単独では治癒を望むことはできず、放射線治療は必須である。発症年齢が低いために、高次脳機能の障害を減らすために照射線量を減らす試みがなされている。照射野は髄液を介した転移を考慮して全脳室照射とする。

髄芽腫は髄膜播種を高頻度に認めることから手術のみでは治癒不能であり、術後の放射線治療は必須である。照射野は全脳全脊髄照射が標準である。

2)頭頸部

機能と形態を温存するためにも放射線治療の役割は大きい。放射線治療は常に考慮すべき治療であり、手術療法から化学放射線療法に置き換わりつつある病態も多い。上咽頭癌では放射線治療はすべての病期にわたり、標準治療である。声門癌のⅠ期は放射線治療単独で発声という機能を温存して9割を越える5年無病生存が得られる疾患であり、標準治療となっている。

3)乳癌

乳房温存術後に放射線治療を施行することにより、乳房内再発率が低下し、生存期間が延長することが臨床試験において証明されており、温存術後の接線照射は標準治療となっている。

4)肺癌

小細胞肺癌と非小細胞肺癌に分けられる。小細胞肺癌の治療の主体は化学療法であるが、放射線治療の感受性が高く、適宜、放射線治療の追加は必要である。Ⅲ期以上の非小細胞肺癌の治療の主体は化学放射線療法である。照射野

の範囲の決定にPETは有用である。I期非小細胞肺癌では定位放射線治療により手術と同等の成績が得られている。

5) 食道癌

手術不能の場合は、化学放射線療法がすべての病期で適応となりうる。

6) 子宮頸癌

日本ではI、II期は切除されることが一般であるが、欧米ではI、II期も放射線治療が行われることが多い。III期、IVa期は放射線治療が第1選択である。外照射と腔内照射の併用が一般で、腔内照射の線量の基準点としてA点が用いられる。A点は外子宮口を原点として子宮腔内に向かって2cm、そこから直角に外側に2cm離れた点である。

7) 悪性リンパ腫

病期I-II期の濾胞性リンパ腫の第一選択は放射線治療である。一般には化学療法（CHOP）後に腫瘍の浸潤範囲に放射線治療を施行する。胃MALTリンパ腫では、ピロリ菌の除菌後に残存を認める場合に照射する。

8) 緩和的放射線治療

放射線治療はうまく使えば緩和治療としても有効である。最も多く用いられているのは骨転移に対する疼痛解除目的の治療である。腫瘍出血に対しての止血にも有効である。

放射線治療の将来

癌の罹患率は年齢とともに急激に上昇し、今後、さまざまな疾患をもった癌患者が急速に増加すると予想される。放射線治療は根治から姑息までのあらゆる状況の治療が可能な低侵襲治療として、その重要性はますます増してくるであろう。

放射線治療の理想は、正常組織に障害を与えることなく、腫瘍に放射線を集中して、非侵襲的に腫瘍を根絶することである。この理想に近づくのに機器の進歩の果たした役割は大きかった。10年ほど前までは、さまざまな照射方法の線量分布シミュレーションを行い、最善の治療法を選択するというのが高度な治療であった。しかし、強度変調放射線治療という

腫瘍に必要な線量を投与し重要臓器には線量制約を設けて、それを実現するための最適解をコンピュータに計算させるという革命的な方法が出現し、放射線治療はさらに理想に近づいた。この治療法は今では一般の放射線治療機にも標準装備され、これに回転照射を加えたVMATも実現し、Tomotherapy、Cyberknife、Veroなどの専用機も登場した。一方で、X線の物理学的限界を超えるために粒子線治療が実用段階に入ろうとしている。今後の発展のひとつは陽子線などの粒子線治療が小型・低価格化して、一般治療化することであろうか。

化学放射線療法の有効性が多くの疾患で示され、標準治療化してきて、腫瘍学のなかにおける放射線治療という考え方が定着してきた。さらに、分子生物学の進歩により多くの分子標的薬剤が出現し、癌治療を根本から変化させる様相を帯びてきた。今後は、適切な分子標的薬の併用にとどまらず、治療効果予測がより正確となって適切な患者選択が可能となってくるであろう。本文にもあるとおり、小細胞肺癌でCRとなった症例には全脳照射を行うのが標準である。これにより、脳内の再発が減るため予防的全脳照射と呼ばれているが、ワクチンのように再発を予防しているわけではない。すなわち、画像で検出できない微小腫瘍が残っているなら画像上に現れてくる前に治療する超早期治療、残っていなかった人には無駄な治療をしたことになる。同様の無駄な治療は前立腺癌、乳癌にもあることが臨床試験の結果から証明できる。今後は、このような治療は少なくなり、分子生物学の知見をもとにより選択された被験者による効率的な臨床試験が行われるようになろう。

このように、放射線治療の枠の中だけにとどまれない時代がすでに来ている。現時点では、無駄な治療となりうる場合には少なくとも有害事象を起こさないことが重要であろう。将来、より適切な患者選択ができるようになれば、無駄な治療がなくなり、さらなる放射線治療の進歩に繋がる。このように、放射線治療の進歩は周辺の進歩に支えられている。広い視野で放射線治療の将来を考える必要があろう。

略　語

GTV: Gross Tumor Volume　肉眼的腫瘍体積
CTV: Clinical Target Volume　臨床標的体積
PTV: Planning Target Volume　計画標的体積

【臨床試験グループ】
EORTC: European Organization for Research and Treatment of Cancer
ECOG: Eastern Cooperative Oncology Group
ESPAC: Eastern Study Group for Pancreatic Cancer
GOG: Gynecologic Oncology Group
JROSG: Japanese Radiation Oncology Study Group
MRC: Medical Research Council
NCCTG: North Central Cancer Treatment Group
NSABP: National Surgical Adjuvant Breast and Bowel Project
NWTSG: National Wilms Tumor Study Group
RTOG: Radiation Therapy Oncology Group
SWOG: Soethwest Oncology Group
NRG: 臨床グループの再編の中で、NSABP、RTOG、GOGがNRGに統合された。

【化学療法レジメ】
ABVD: Adriamycin, Bleomycin, Vinblastine, Dacarbazine
CHOP: Cyclophosphamide, Hydroxydaunorubicine, Oncovin, Predonine
MOPP: Mechlorethamine, Oncovin, Procarbazine, Predonine

執筆者一覧

[監修]
中山秀次（東京医科大学 放射線医学分野 准教授）
德植公一（東京医科大学 放射線医学分野 主任教授）

執筆者（東京医科大学 放射線医学分野）
糸永知弘〔後期研修医〕
　3.胸部（2～4）／13.参考資料
大久保充〔講師〕
　1.中枢神経／4.消化器（5～7）／5.泌尿器
齋藤辰彦〔後期研修医〕
　8.緩和
白石沙眞〔助教〕
　6.婦人科癌／12.良性疾患
菅原信二〔教授〕
　10.骨軟部腫瘍／11.小児
田島　祐〔助教〕
　2.頭頸部／4.消化器（2～4）／13.参考資料
德植公一〔主任教授〕
　13.参考資料
德増健二〔後期研修医〕
　8.緩和
中山秀次〔准教授〕
　7.血液・リンパ腫
三上隆二〔講師〕
　3.胸部（1）／4.消化器（1）／9.皮膚癌

新・放射線治療ポケットマニュアル

2015(平成27)年11月16日　初版第1刷発行
定価　本体1,500円(税別)

編著者	中山秀次
	徳植公一
発行人	分部康平
発行所	産業開発機構株式会社
	〒111-0053
	東京都台東区浅草橋2-2-10 カナレビル
	TEL　03-3861-7051
	FAX　03-5687-7744
	http://www.eizojoho.co.jp/
	郵便振込　00110-2-14817
印刷	株式会社フォレスト

＊禁・無断転載
ISBN　978-86028-225-7 C3047　￥1500E